Military Use of Drugs
Not Yet Approved by the FDA
for CW/BW Defense

Military Use of Drugs Not Yet Approved by the FDA for CW/BW Defense

LESSONS FROM THE GULF WAR

Richard A. Rettig

Prepared for the Office of the Secretary of Defense

National Defense Research Institute

RAND

This report is one of several commissioned by the Special Assistant to the Deputy Secretary of Defense for Gulf War Illnesses. It deals with the Interim Rule, adopted in December 1990, which established the authority of the Commissioner of Food and Drugs to waive informed consent for using investigational drugs in certain military contingencies. The contingency for which it was adopted and in which it was used was the 1991 Gulf War, when U.S. and coalition forces confronted the possibility of chemical and biological weapons being used by the Iraqi military. The investigational drugs in question were pyridostigmine bromide and botulinum toxoid vaccine.

In mid-1997, when the research on which this report is based was completed, the rule making initiated by the Interim Rule had not been completed. Rule making resumed, however, with the issuance on July 31, 1997 of a "Request for Comments" by the Food and Drug Administration (FDA) (62 *Federal Register* 40996), "Accessibility to New Drugs for Use in Military and Civilian Exigencies When Traditional Human Efficacy Studies are Not Feasible; Determination Under the Interim Rule That Informed Consent Is Not Feasible for Military Exigencies." This request asked for public comment on the merits of issuing an unchanged Interim Rule as a final rule, modifying the current rule, or revoking it entirely. Although comments were received in response to this FDA request, rule making had not been completed by summer 1998. However, by mid-October, Congress resolved the issue with the enactment of Sec. 731 of the Strom Thurmond National Defense Authorization Act for Fiscal Year 1999 (Public Law 105-261, October 17, 1998). This statutory enactment vested the authority to grant waivers, initially authorized by the Interim Rule, solely in the President of the United States. A brief postscript at the end of this report summarizes these developments.

This long lapse of time between the adoption of the Interim Rule and the statutory resolution of policy issues raised by it reflects both the low frequency with which the threat of chemical and biological weapons arises and the complexity of the issues raised by the rule. Regarding the frequency, Judge Ruth

Bader Ginsburg, then the circuit court judge for the U.S. Court of Appeals for the District of Columbia Circuit, wrote in 1991 that the likelihood of U.S. military personnel encountering chemical and biological warfare threats in the future fell "in the middle ground between cases in which the recurrence prospect is nonexistent or extremely remote, and those in which the probability of repetition is extremely high."[1] Such uncertain threats with potentially disastrous consequences pose difficult challenges for both military and civilian policymakers. This report attempts to contribute to the understanding of the complexity of the issues surrounding the Interim Rule and to an understanding of the controversy that was only recently resolved.

The other RAND reports are reviews of the scientific literature on the health effects of chemical and biological agents, pyridostigmine bromide, oil fire pollution, depleted uranium, pesticides, infectious diseases, immunizations, and stress.

This work is sponsored by the Office of the Special Assistant and was carried out jointly by RAND Health's Center for Military Health Policy Research and the Forces and Resources Policy Center of the National Defense Research Institute. The latter is a federally funded research and development center sponsored by the Office of the Secretary of Defense, the Joint Staff, the unified commands and the defense agencies.

The audiences for whom this paper is intended include the civilian and military officials responsible for doctrine, policy, and systems related to the deployment of troops to theaters of operation where the threat of attack with chemical and biological weapons is a real possibility, including those responsible for the protection of the health and fitness of U.S. military personnel and for the conduct of supporting medical research and drug development. Another audience is the civilian officials responsible for administering the laws and regulations governing the review and approval of drugs and vaccines for military use, including those officials with specific responsibilities for the protection of human subjects of research. Finally, a critical audience is the American public concerned that its public policies regarding the protection and treatment of U.S. military personnel deployed to hostile environments in which they face the threat of chemical or biological weapons are simultaneously pragmatic and ethical.

---

[1] *Doe v. Sullivan*, 938 F2nd 1370, No. 91-5019, USApp DC 111, heard March 18, 1991, decided July 16, 1991.

CONTENTS

FIGURE AND TABLES

Figure

Tables

In August 1990, after Iraq invaded neighboring Kuwait, the United States government mobilized for potential conflict. Operation Desert Shield, in the fall of 1990, involved troop mobilization and force deployment; concurrently, Congress debated the wisdom of going to war with Iraq. Operation Desert Shield, the actual combat in the Gulf, occurred between mid-January and late February 1991, with the coalition forces decisively defeating the Iraqi military.

One threat the United States faced in the Gulf War was that Iraq might use chemical warfare (CW) and/or biological warfare (BW) agents. The Department of Defense's (DoD's) defensive measures against CW/BW weapons, imperfect as they are, included detection, protection, and medical measures (including both prophylactic and therapeutic interventions).

Several medical products were available to DoD for potential defensive and prophylactic use in response to CW and BW attacks. But the FDA had not approved these products for these indications. Thus, the FDA regulatory framework designated these products as investigational new drugs (INDs). Pyridostigmine bromide (PB), a drug for pretreatment against certain nerve agents, had been approved long ago for the treatment of myasthenia gravis in larger doses and for longer times than the anticipated Gulf War use. Thus, there was a *prima facie* case for safety based on experience in humans; there were also animal studies that supported its effectiveness. Botulinum toxin (BT) was a vaccine used routinely in occupational settings in which workers were at risk of botulism. Both the U.S. Army and the Centers for Disease Control also registered BT as an IND.

DoD wished to be in a position to use PB and BT, if necessary, but also wished to act either in compliance with FDA regulations governing INDs or with formal FDA concurrence that it could act without FDA approval. DoD and FDA recognized that neither DoD statutory or administrative authority nor the federal Food, Drug, and Cosmetic Act (FDCA) or its implementing regulations had been written with the contingency of the Gulf War in mind. The DoD-FDA discussions foreclosed the possibility of DoD action independent of FDA. This led DoD to request that FDA waive informed consent and other requirements of the IND regulations. Consequently, after several months of discussion, and within weeks of active combat, the Secretary of Health and Human Services and the Commissioner of Food and Drugs jointly issued an Interim Rule establishing the authority of the Commissioner to waive IND requirements in certain military exigencies (55 FR 52814, December 21, 1990).

The provisions of the Interim Rule included the following:

- The Commissioner of Food and Drugs could determine that informed consent was "not feasible" at the request of the Assistant Secretary of Defense (Health Affairs) in connection with "the use of an investigational drug . . . in a specific protocol" under an IND sponsored by DoD.

- The DoD request must be limited to a specific military situation involving "combat or the immediate threat of combat."

- The request must include written justification supporting the conclusions

  > that a military combat exigency exists because of special military combat (actual or threatened) circumstances in which, in order to facilitate the accomplishment of the military mission, preservation of the health of the individual and the safety of other personnel require that a particular treatment be provided to a specified group of military personnel, without regard to what might be any individual's personal preference for no treatment or for some alternative treatment.

- The waiver request must have been reviewed by a duly constituted institutional review board

- The Commissioner's decision must be based on a finding that obtaining informed consent is not feasible and that "withholding treatment would be contrary to the best interests of military personnel and there is no available satisfactory alternative therapy."

In reaching his decision, the Commissioner must take into account

1. the "extent and strength of the evidence of the safety and effectiveness of the investigational drug for the intended use"

2. the context in which the drug would be administered

3. the nature of the disease or condition for which preventive or therapeutic treatment is intended

4. the information to be provided to the recipients regarding the "potential benefits and risks of taking or not taking the drug."

The Commissioner, in reaching his determination, is authorized to consult appropriate experts. A waiver of informed consent resulting from a determination by the Commissioner would expire after 12 months, unless renewed, or when DoD informs the Commissioner that the conflict has ceased, whichever comes earlier. After the issuance of the Interim Rule, DoD requested time-limited waivers for PB and BT, which FDA granted in early January 1991.

The DoD Gulf War experience in the use of PB and BT was characterized by poor record keeping, inadequate data collection, and other violations of the terms agreed to in the FDA waivers. This experience raised questions for FDA about the DoD's ability to administer the waivers and, for the critics of the Interim Rule, called the wisdom of the rule itself into question.

After the war, many Gulf War veterans reported a number of poorly diagnosed illnesses. A variety of hypotheses have been advanced regarding the exposure of military personnel to various chemical, biological, and environmental agents and the possible relationship between these exposures and the veterans' reported illnesses. PB and BT were among the agents that some, especially veterans, believed to have caused some of the Gulf War veterans' illnesses. The above factors, especially poor administration and the hypothesized (although not supported by data) relationships between the PB and BT and Gulf War veterans' illnesses, deterred FDA completion of the rule-making process.

The completion of rule making regarding the Interim Rule has taken a very complicated course in the eight years since the rule's issuance. First, the U.S. District Court of the District of Columbia upheld the rule on the grounds that the issue was not reviewable but that, if it were, the court would defer to the administrative agency implementing the rule (*John Doe and Mary Doe v. Louis Sullivan and Richard Cheney*, USDC, District of Columbia, 756F. Suppl. 12, January 31, 1991). The U.S. Circuit Court of Appeals for the District of Columbia, on appeal, held that the issue was reviewable, but that FDA acted within its authority in issuing the rule (*Doe v. Sullivan*, 938 F.2d 1370, No. 91-5019, USApp DC 111, July 16, 1991). In early 1991, then, FDA was ready to proceed to a final rule, especially after the courts upheld the Commissioner's authority. However, other, more normal, FDA priorities asserted themselves after the Gulf War ended, and delay set in. The emergence of sharply differing points of view within FDA on the merits of the Interim Rule reinforced the delay.

Second, the Presidential Advisory Committee (PAC) on Gulf War Veterans' Illnesses, formed in late 1995 and operating in 1996 and 1997, in its *Interim Report* (PAC, 1996b), its *Final Report* (PAC, 1996c), and in a letter report subsequent to the *Final Report*, recommended completion of the rule-making process. The PAC did not take a position on the controversial substantive issues surrounding the Interim Rule but did criticize DoD's implementation of the rule in the actual combat situation.

Third, FDA, prodded by successive recommendations of the PAC, published a request for comments on the merits of the Interim Rule in mid-1997, asking that respondents address the options of issuing it as a final rule, modifying it, or revoking it entirely (62 FR 40996, July 31, 1996). This published request was an antecedent action before FDA published its own proposed final rule. By mid-1998, it was known that FDA had proposed to revoke the authority the Interim Rule established, that DoD had objected to revocation, and that the matter was under discussion at the Office of Management and Budget (OMB).

Finally, in the summer of 1998, language (known as the Byrd amendment) was inserted into the Defense Authorization Act for Fiscal Year 1999 that would have required the Secretary of Defense to submit waiver requests, with the written concurrence of the President and with notification of the relevant congressional committees (S. 2057, July 20, 1998). Previously, under the Interim Rule, the Assistant Secretary of Defense (Health Affairs) was to submit such requests. The proposed legislation assumed the continuance of the Interim Rule, at least in some form. However, FDA revocation of the rule would nullify the effect of the legislation, because no one would have the authority to receive such a request. Consequently, the legislation actually adopted in October 1998 (Sec. 731, National Defense Authorization Act for Fiscal Year 1999, Public Law 105-261, October 17, 1998) modified the original language from the summer and vested the authority to grant waivers solely in the President of the United States. The criteria to be used in granting the waivers were the same as those of the Interim Rule. Hence, the policy conflict was resolved by statute, and OMB told the FDA and DoD to resolve their differences within the frame of the new legislation. That process is now under way.

This report reviews the history of the Interim Rule, including the deliberations between DoD and FDA in late 1990, the litigation that occurred in 1991, the actual Gulf War experience with PB and BT, and the work of the PAC. It also addresses the substantive issues raised by the Interim Rule, especially the ethical questions surrounding the waiver of informed consent as authorized by the Interim Rule. It then analyzes the issues FDA outlined in its 1997 request for comments (62 FR 40996, July 31, 1996), including the independence of the investigational review board in reviewing waiver requests, the determination that informed consent is "not feasible" in certain combat situations, the information about investigational drugs that is provided to military personnel in Gulf War–like situations, record keeping, procedures to track noncompliance, and alternatives to the Interim Rule. The report also discusses the question of authority stemming from the absence in the Constitution, in DoD statutes and regulations, and in the FDCA and its regulations of provisions for a contingency of the Gulf War type.

This report was written before the Byrd amendment was proposed and adopted. Therefore, although it refers to these legislative developments, the analysis of the Interim Rule reflects the issues as they were presented in 1997.

ACKNOWLEDGMENTS

A number of individuals provided assistance in obtaining documents and other information and in explaining some of the complex arguments associated with the subject of this report.

In the Department of Defense: Gary Christopherson, Office of the Assistant Secretary of Defense (Health Affairs), organized a briefing for the RAND group involved in the Gulf War study in the fall of 1996. He also listened to a briefing of this study in October 1997 and made useful criticisms at that time. John Casciotti, Office of the General Counsel, DoD, was very generous with his time in two lengthy interviews. Ronald E. Clawson, Project Manager, Pharmaceutical Systems, U.S. Army Medical Materiel Development Activity, organized a half-day meeting with his senior staff in spring 1997 to explain pyridostigmine bromide and botulinum toxoid, provided useful background documents and organized a briefing in January 1998 for his staff. Edmund Howe, a physician and lawyer at the Uniformed Services University of Health Sciences, discussed the ethics of the Interim Rule in a 1997 interview.

In the Food and Drug Administration, Stuart Nightingale, Associate Commissioner for Health Affairs, and Brian Malkin, Office of Health Affairs, provided documents and arranged a meeting with Mary Pendergast, Deputy Commissioner; Robert Temple, Center for Drug Evaluation and Research; and Karen Goldenthal, Center for Biologics Evaluation and Research.

In addition, Charles McCarthy, former director, Office for the Protection of Research Risks, Department of Health and Human Services, in a lengthy telephone interview, recalled the discussion that occurred in the fall of 1990 associated with the Interim Rule. Joan Porter, professional staff of the Presidential Advisory Committee on Gulf War Veterans' Illnesses, was helpful in several interviews, in providing useful background information, and in arranging an interview with Robyn Nishimi, Staff Director of the committee.

The two reviewers of this report made helpful criticisms that improved the final product. I take full responsibility for any remaining problems of fact or interpretation.

2-PAM	Pralidoxime chloride, one of the two antidotes for nerve agents
ACHRE	Advisory Committee on Human Radiation Experiments
ASD(HA)	Assistant Secretary of Defense (Health Affairs)
Atropine	Atropine sulfate, one of the two antidotes for nerve agents
AX	Vaccine against anthrax
BLA	Biologic Licensing Application
BT	The botulinum toxoid vaccine
BW	Biological warfare
CBER	Center for Biologics Evaluation and Research
CBW	Chemical and biological warfare
CDER	Center for Drug Evaluation and Research
CENTCOM	U.S. Central Command
CFR	Code of Federal Regulations
CINCCENT	Commander in Chief, U.S. Central Command
CW	Chemical warfare
DHHS	Department of Health and Human Services
DoD	Department of Defense
ELA	Establishment Licensing Application
FDA	Food and Drug Administration
FDCA	Food, Drug, and Cosmetic Act
FORSCOM	U.S. Army Forces Command
FR	*Federal Register*
HIV	Human immunodeficiency virus

HSRRB	The Army Surgeon General's Human Subjects Research Review Board
HURRAD	Human Use Review and Regulatory Affairs Division
ICWRG	Informed Consent Waiver Review Group
IDE	Investigational device exemption
IND	Investigational new drug
IOM	Institute of Medicine
IRB	Institutional review board
JAMA	*Journal of the American Medical Association*
MOU	Memorandum of understanding
NDA	New Drug Application
NIH	National Institutes of Health
NPRM	Notice of Proposed Rule Making
ODS	Operation Desert Shield/Desert Storm
OGC	Office of the General Counsel
OMB	Office of Management and Budget
OPRR	Office for Protection from Research Risks
PAC	Presidential Advisory Committee on Gulf War Veterans' Illnesses
PB	Pyridostigmine bromide, pretreatment for exposure to nerve agents
PGVCB	Persian Gulf Veterans Coordinating Board
PLA	Product Licensing Application
TBE	Tick-borne encephalitis
UNSCOM	United Nations Special Commission
USC	United States Code
VX	A nerve agent that can be absorbed through lungs and skin

Chapter One

INTRODUCTION

PURPOSE AND ORGANIZATION

This report examines the regulatory issues associated with the use of drugs not yet approved by the Federal Food and Drug Administration (FDA) for the defense of military forces against chemical and biological warfare agents. It uses the 1991 Gulf War as the point of departure but deals with the issues in the context of contemporary FDA policymaking.

The purposes of this report are (1) to examine historically the adoption in 1990, in the shadow of the impending Gulf War, of the Interim Rule (55 FR 52814, December 21, 1990), which authorized the Commissioner of Food and Drugs to waive informed consent for the use of investigational drugs and vaccines for certain military uses; how this authority was used for pyridostigmine bromide and botulinum toxoid; and the subsequent controversy surrounding the rule, its application, and its implications; (2) to analyze the issues the Interim Rule raised when investigational drugs are used for such purposes; and (3) to make recommendations.

Chapter Two examines the historical development of the Interim Rule. Chapter Three addresses the definitional issues surrounding *investigational*. In Chapter Four, the Interim Rule and its alternatives are considered. Chapter Five discusses several broader issues than the immediate regulatory questions the Interim Rule itself raised. Finally, in Chapter Six, conclusions are drawn and recommendations are made.

BACKGROUND

The Iraqi Threat

Iraq invaded Kuwait on August 2, 1990. In response, the U.S. government demanded its withdrawal, deployed over half a million military personnel to Saudi Arabia (Operation Desert Shield) to deter further Iraqi aggression against neighboring states, and initiated a United Nations debate that called for Iraq's withdrawal by January 15. When Iraq ignored this deadline, coalition forces, led by the U.S. military, initiated active conflict in the early AM hours of January 17. In Operation Desert Storm,[1] coalition forces quickly overwhelmed Iraqi forces; after six weeks, in late February, President Bush halted military operations.[2]

It was well known that the Iraqi military capability included *both* chemical warfare and biological warfare (CW/BW) agents. This threat was well publicized to U.S. troops deployed to Saudi Arabia and has since been confirmed in detail in 1995 and later the United Nations Special Commission (UNSCOM).

The CW threat by Iraq was the most serious since the use of mustard gas in World War I. Iraq had used CW agents in its war with Iran as well as against its own citizens. There are four types of CW agents: nerve, vesicant, blood, and pulmonary agents. Nerve agents are organophosphorous inhibitors of acetylcholinesterase; vesicants are skin-blistering compounds, such as mustards and arsenicals; and blood agents are the cyanides, inhibitors of cytochrome oxidase. (Keeler et al., 1991). Pulmonary agents, such as chlorine, phosgene, and diphosgene, irritate the eyes and injure the respiratory system and may cause pulmonary edema. (Sidell, Takafuji, and Franz, 1997.)

The Iraqi CW arsenal was believed to include nerve, vesicant, and blood agents (Keeler et al., 1991), but the primary threat was that of nerve agents. Nerve agents are effective for CW because they are extremely potent inhibitors of the enzyme acetylcholinesterase, a key regulator of cholinergic neurotransmission in tissue. When this enzyme is severely inhibited, the resulting buildup of acetylcholine is fatal. Nerve agents include three inhalation "G" agents—tabun, sarin, and soman—and VX, which can be absorbed through both the lungs and the skin. (Dunn and Sidell, 1989). G agents, which are liquids at moderate temperatures, are typically distributed by droplets or aerosol and evaporate and disperse over several hours under temperate conditions. Tabun, sarin, and soman are "nonpersistent." VX, an oily liquid, is persistent.

The Iraqi BW threat included anthrax, which is caused by a powerful and highly toxic microorganism, *Bacillus anthracis*, and botulism, a neurotoxin (botulinum toxin), which is produced by the bacterium *Clostridium botulinum*. Both are capable of inducing lethal effects to exposed humans and animals. The protective measures against these biological agents include vaccines—AX vaccine against anthrax and botulinum toxoid (BT) against botulism.

Both before and during ODS, the Department of Defense (DoD) gave substantial attention to countermeasures for protecting troops against CW/BW attack

---

[1]The abbreviation ODS will be used throughout to refer to both Operation Desert Shield and Operation Desert Storm; the specific meaning will be clear in context.

[2]Desert Storm involved 41 days of intensive bombing in the air campaign and 100 hours of a ground attack. (Scales, 1993.)

and maintaining military effectiveness. Protection against nerve agent exposure includes detection and warning devices, use of chemical protective masks and protective clothing, and medical management. Medical management of nerve agent exposure involves a three-drug regimen: pretreatment with pyridostigmine bromide (PB) before exposure and administration of two antidotes, atropine sulfate (Atropine) and pralidoxime chloride (2-PAM), intramuscularly by autoinjectors after actual exposure. (The antidotes are components of the Mark I Nerve Agent Antidote Kit.) The rationale for the use of PB as a *pretreatment* for anticipated nerve agent exposure is that it temporarily (i.e., reversibly) occupies the same tissue receptor sites as does nerve agent, thus blocking the nerve agent from permanently inhibiting acetylcholinesterase and achieving lethal effects. The blocking action of PB allows *treatment* by atropine, which blocks the effects of excess acetylcholine, and pralidoxime chloride, which pulls the nerve agent off acetylcholinesterase. In short, PB pretreatment is indicated because it offers sufficient protection against rapid-acting nerve agent to permit therapy to be administered.

The Regulatory Regime

The Food Drug and Cosmetic Act (FDCA) vests authority in the Secretary of Health and Human Services, who then delegates it to the Commissioner of Food and Drugs, to regulate the development, testing, and evaluation of drugs, biologics (including vaccines), and medical devices, and other matters.[3] The FDCA prohibits the introduction of a drug into interstate commerce until it has been approved by FDA as "safe for use" and "effective in use." Approval may be revoked if a drug is subsequently found to be unsafe for use or not effective in use.

The *safety* of a drug is to be based on "adequate tests by all methods reasonably applicable." [Sec. 505(d)(1), FDCA] The *effectiveness* of a drug is to be based on "substantial evidence that the drug will have the effect it purports or is repre-

---

[3]Under the FDCA, as amended [Ch. 2, Sec. 201[321](g)(1)], the term *drug* means

> (A) articles recognized in the official United States Pharmacopoeia, official Homeopathic Pharmacopoeia of the United States, or official National Formulary, or any supplement to any of them; and (B) articles intended for use in the diagnosis, cure, mitigation, treatment, or prevention of disease in man or other animals; and (C) articles (other than food) intended to affect the structure or any function of the body of many or other animals; and (D) articles intended for use as a component of any articles specified in clause (A), (B), or (C); but does not included devices or their components, parts, or accessories."

Biological products, including vaccines, are defined as "any virus, therapeutic serum, toxin, antitoxin, or analogous product applicable to the prevention, treatment, or cure of diseases or injuries of man." [21 Code of Federal Regulations (CFR) Part 600, § 600.3(h)] For purposes of evaluating safety and effectiveness, the term *drug* applies both to drugs (usually chemical entities) and to biological products, also known as biologics. Drugs and biologics are regulated in basically the same way; devices are regulated somewhat differently; the distinction does not concern us in this report.

sented to have under the conditions of use prescribed, recommended, or suggested in the proposed labeling thereof." [Sec. 505(d)(5), FDCA] *Substantial evidence* is defined as

> evidence consisting of adequate and well-controlled investigations, including clinical investigations, by experts qualified by scientific training and experience to evaluate the effectiveness of the drug involved, on the basis of which it could fairly and responsibly be concluded by such experts that the drug will have the effect it purports or is represented to have under the conditions of use prescribed, recommended, or suggested in the labeling or proposed labeling thereof. [Sec. 505(d)]

Under the law, the Secretary of Health and Human Services is required to issue regulations *exempting* those drugs "intended solely for *investigational use* [emphasis added] by experts qualified by scientific training and experience to investigate the safety and effectiveness of drugs" from the regulations applying to approved drugs. These regulations require that an investigational new drug (IND) application[4] be filed with FDA by the sponsor of a drug or biologic "before any clinical testing of a new drug is undertaken"; that sponsors agree on supervision of investigators, record keeping, and filing of reports; and that written *informed consent* be obtained from individual subjects (or patients) receiving such drugs. IND regulations govern the initial studies of toxicity or safety (Phase I clinical trials) and later studies of effectiveness (Phase II and Phase III trials).

When a sponsor[5] of a drug or biologic concludes that the evidence of safety and effectiveness from well-controlled studies (Phase III) is adequate to secure FDA approval for marketing, a New Drug Application (NDA) is submitted for a drug, or a Product Licensing Application (PLA) and an Establishment Licensing Application (ELA) are submitted for a biologic.[6] FDA then evaluates the NDA, or the PLA/ELA, and either approves or disapproves the application. FDA approval means that the drug or biologic in question satisfies the criteria of being safe and effective and, therefore, may be sold and promoted in interstate commerce *for the specific use or indication* the FDA approved. FDA approval

---

[4]Technically, an Investigational New Drug (IND) is an *application* to the FDA for approval to conduct clinical investigations related to the safety and effectiveness of a drug or biologic. The term is also used to refer to an investigational *drug* that is being tested in humans under an FDA-approved IND. The meaning in this report will be clear in the context of its use.

[5]Sponsors of Phase III drugs and biologics are usually, but not always, commercial drug firms; sponsors of Phase I and Phase II studies often include academic institutions and investigators as well.

[6]As one aspect of Reinventing Government, the PLA and ELA distinction was eliminated in 1997 in favor of a Biologic Licensing Application (BLA), which includes both product and establishment considerations and is consistent with the NDA nomenclature for drugs.

also carries with it other requirements, such as product labeling, manufacturing quality control, reporting of adverse effects, and sponsor advertising.

For drugs not yet approved, but used in clinical trials that are designed to obtain evidence for approval, FDA has established regulations regarding informed consent. The FDCA requires that "experts using . . . drugs for investigational purposes" certify to the sponsor of such investigations

> that they will inform any human beings to whom such drugs, or any controls used therewith, are being administered, or their representatives, that such drugs are being used for investigational purposes and will obtain the consent of such human beings or their representatives, except where they deem it not feasible or, in their professional judgment, contrary to the best interests of such human beings. [Sec. 505(I)(3), FDCA]

Specific FDA informed consent requirements implement this statutory language. In addition, FDA requirements conform to the Department of Health and Human Services (DHHS) informed consent regulations for the clinical research of the National Institutes of Health (NIH) and the Centers for Disease Control (CDC) (45 CFR 46); and to the "Common Rule." The last regulation applies to all federal agencies and requires that an Institutional Review Board (IRB) review and approve research protocols involving human subjects according to the following criteria: (1) risks to subjects are minimized; (2) risks to subjects are reasonable in relation to anticipated benefits; (3) selection of subjects is equitable; (4) informed consent will be sought from each subject in accordance with the general requirements for informed consent; (5) informed consent will be appropriately documented; (6) when appropriate, provision will be made for monitoring the data collected to ensure safety of subjects; and (7) when appropriate, provisions will be made to ensure privacy and confidentiality of subject data.

The Drugs in Question

It is important to emphasize that FDA's classification of a drug as investigational or licensed is *use-specific*. Of the three entities considered in this report—PB, AX, and BT—only AX vaccine was an FDA *licensed* drug for a use or indication comparable to its likely use in the Gulf War, i.e., as an effective vaccine against inhaled anthrax. Thus, it was available for DoD use without any requirements applicable to investigational drugs.

PB is *licensed* for two civilian uses. It was first synthesized in 1945 and, after extensive testing, was approved (i.e., licensed) by FDA in 1955 as safe for the treatment of myasthenia gravis (NDA No. 9829, April 7, 1955). Produced by Hoffman-LaRoche, it is prescribed as Mestinon for this indication for lifetime use and at average daily dosages as much as six times greater than those used in the Gulf War for nerve agent pretreatment. FDA has also approved PB for use in reversing some of the effects of some anesthetic formulations. In this form, it is known as Regenol.

However, today as in 1990, the FDA considers PB to be *investigational* for prophylactic use against CW agents. PB had not been approved as a pretreatment against nerve agents on the eve of the Gulf War, although it had been under investigation for such a use since the U.S. Army filed an IND application with the FDA in 1984 (IND No. 23509, March 1984). The proposed addition of the drug to the U.S. therapeutic regime as a pretreatment for nerve agent poisoning was based on supporting studies conducted in the 1980s and earlier (Dunn and Sidell, 1989). The *safety* of PB for military use had been established on the basis of many well-controlled animal and human studies, including 25 studies in five different animal species in single doses and for as long as 34 weeks. But claims about the *effectiveness* of PB as a pretreatment were based solely on animal studies. The reason for this is clear. It is unethical to expose individuals to lethal nerve agents in order to test the effectiveness of a pretreatment. The United States decided to stock PB tablets (30 mg) in 1986 as a wartime contingency pretreatment (Dunn and Sidell, 1989).

FDA also classified the BT vaccine as investigational at the time of the Gulf War, and this classification remains so today. BT vaccine has been used routinely since the 1980s by individuals in certain agricultural occupations at risk of botulism under an IND held by the Centers for Disease Control (Bureau of Biologics IND #161, November 23, 1965). Although this use of the vaccine is likely to continue, the threat of botulism is infrequent and a significant market for BT vaccine does not exist. Thus, it is unlikely to attract a commercial sponsor and will probably remain in an unlicensed, and therefore investigational status indefinitely.[7] Again, as with PB, the FDA has not approved the BT vaccine for prophylactic use against botulism in the case of a BW attack. Thus, since there are no specific FDA-licensed uses for the BT vaccine, its distribution and use are governed by the regulations that apply to investigational drugs.

However, the meaning of the term *investigational* requires clarification. It is a legal term FDA uses to distinguish between licensed and unlicensed drugs. Although there are scientific bases for the term, *investigational* is not synony-

---

[7]A major reason these drugs remain investigational, although not the only one, is that FDA requires human efficacy data for approval of drugs. Obtaining such data for drugs intended for prophylactic use against CW/BW agents has been regarded as unjustifiable on the ethical grounds that it would involve exposing human beings to lethal doses of such agents, then determining the effectiveness of the prophylactic and therapeutic drugs in question to prevent death or serious injury. The issue raised by this prohibition has been how to evaluate drugs intended for CW/BW defense. However, in July 1997, FDA asked whether there were scientific and ethical ways "to expose volunteers to toxic chemical and biological agents to test the effectiveness of products that may be used to provide potential protection against those agents?" [62 FR 41001, July 29, 1997] This question is discussed in Chapter Four, with respect to Question B.

mous with *experimental*, even though it is often used in that way by many commentators. Normally, informed consent is required in advance for the use of investigational drugs, whereas this is not an FDA requirement for FDA-approved drugs.

The Response to the Iraqi Threat

In response to the Iraqi CW/BW threat, DoD concluded that it needed to be prepared to use PB and BT, and possibly other investigational drugs and medical devices (see Table 1), for defense against potential CW and BW threats, that it should seek FDA approval for using these investigational products for treatment or pretreatment purposes, and that obtaining informed consent of service members in ODS was not feasible. Therefore, on October 30, 1990, DoD requested FDA to establish authority to waive the requirement of informed consent for the use of investigational drugs in certain military exigencies.

FDA responded to this request by issuing an Interim Rule, published in the *Federal Register* on December 21, 1990, "Informed consent for human drugs and biologics; determination that informed consent is not feasible for military exigencies," (55 FR 52814, 1991).[8] Under this rule, DoD then requested waivers of the informed consent requirement for two investigational drugs: PB and BT. These were granted on January 8, 1991.

The Interim Rule, which became effective immediately, did not go unchallenged. Concurrently, FDA also requested public comments on it, of which many were favorable but some were quite opposed. The rule was also contested in the U.S. District Court for the District of Columbia in January 1991 (*Doe v. Sullivan*, 1991). Judge Stanley S. Harris, ruled against a request for a preliminary injunction filed by John Doe, a service member in the Gulf War, and Mary Doe, his wife, on the grounds that this was not a reviewable issue for the courts, and, if it were, Harris would reject the request on its merits. Harris granted the U.S. government's motion to dismiss. The ruling was upheld in July 1991 by the U.S. Circuit Court of Appeals for the District of Columbia, stating the matter to be reviewable but upholding the government on the merits of its case. Some critical commentary also appeared in the popular press and the medical and bioethics literature in early 1991. But by and large, the rule occasioned only limited comment.

After active conflict ended in the spring of 1991, DoD asked FDA to complete the rule-making process and convert the Interim Rule to a final rule. Although

---

[8]The text of the Interim Rule appears at the end of this chapter.

Table 1

Medical Products Under IND Regulation Required or Under Consideration for Use in or Support of ODS, August–September 1990

List Date	Category, Product	IND #, Sponsor	Manufacturer	IND Listed Indication	ODS Status	Scheduled Availability
	Drug products	**IND #**				
8/31/90 9/19/90	Diazepam autoinjector	33,358 USA OTSG	Duphar BV Amsterdam, Netherlands	Preventing nerve agent induced convulsions	Immediate requirement	9/26/90 On schedule
8/31/90 9/19/90	Ribavirin injection	16,666 USA OTSG	Viratech	Hemorrhagic fever with renal syndrome	Immediate requirement	10/7/90
8/31/90 9/19/90	Atropine sulphate inhalation aerosol	27,594 3M Pharmaceuticals NDA# 20-056 USA OTSG	3M Riker developed product; mfr for gov't TBD	Anticholinergic antidote for organophosphate poisoning	Decision pending	5–11 weeks after decision to procure
8/31/90 9/19/90	Pyridostigmine bromide 30 mg tablets	ANDA# 89-572 Kalipharma USA OTSG	Duphar BV Amsterdam, Netherlands	ANDA for myasthenia gravis; for ODS, pretreatment nerve agent	On site per 1983 letter (classified); contract to Duphar for more	9/21/90
9/19/90	Multi Shield	Reg. status under FDA review; mfr has asked reclassification from cosmetic to device	Interpro, Inc., Haverill, MA	ODS topical skin protectant	Procurement under consideration	2 weeks after decision to procure
	Biologic products	**#BB-IND**				
8/31/90 9/19/90	Hepatitis A vaccine inactivated	3200 Smith-Kline-Beecham; 3252, Merck	Smith-Kline-Beecham; Merck	Prevent disease caused by Hep A virus	Not an immediate requirement	Pending, undeter-mined
8/31/90 9/19/90	Botulinal toxoid	161, CDC	Michigan Dept of Public Health	Active immunization against botulism	Immediate requirement	10/1/90
8/31/90 9/19/90	J-5 monoclonal antibody (Centoxin)	2283, Centocor	Centocor	Treatment of septic patients	Immediate requirement	9/10/90

Table 1—Continued

List Date	Category, Product	IND #, Sponsor	Manufacturer	IND Listed Indication	ODS Status	Scheduled Availability
	Device products	**510(k) #**				
9/19/90	Field medical oxygen generating and distribution system	K903411 Guild Associates, Inc.	Guild Associates, Inc.	Produce medical grade oxygen	No immediate requirement	5 prototype on call for shipment to Saudi Arabia
9/19/90	Litter, folding, rigid pole, decontam-ination	K901760 USA MMDA	Arizona Industries for the Blind	Evacuate and decontamin-ate chemical casualties	Immediate requirement	Production of 720 completed; 800 more being procured
9/19/90	Drawover anesthesia device	K901117A USA MMDA	Ohmeda	Deliver anesthetic drugs in field medical units	Immediate requirement for 15 units	
9/19/90	Liquid oxygen system, Genox Model CT-1	K904002 USA OTSG	Pacific Consolidated Industries	Produce medical grade oxygen	2 systems on site; 2 more may be procured	

SOURCE: Department of Defense (1990)

apparently disposed to do so initially, FDA did not act immediately. As the Gulf War receded in public consciousness, the urgency associated with rule making also receded, and differences of view emerged within FDA about the appropriate course of action. FDA had not completed rule making by February 1996, when the Presidential Advisory Committee on Gulf War Veterans' Illnesses (PAC) issued its *Interim Report*. The PAC urged the FDA to complete the rule-making process, a suggestion it repeated in its *Final Report* of December 1996.

Then, in late July 1997, FDA announced plans to complete the rule-making process with publication of a "Request for Comments" on the Interim Rule (62 FR 40996, July 31, 1997). In testimony to the PAC on July 29, then–Deputy Commissioner Mary Pendergast indicated that the agency was also considering a public meeting in early 1998 that would focus on specific issues highlighted by the comments (Pendergast, 1997). She also stated that FDA expected to issue a Notice of Proposed Rule Making (NPRM) in the first half of 1998 after analyzing the comments received. The NPRM would propose a final rule that would modify or revoke the Interim Rule. Thus, resolution of the legal, regulatory, and ethical issues associated with the Interim Rule may occur within the not-too-distant future.[9]

THE ISSUES

The Interim Rule raised three sets of issues. The first set involves contextual issues pertaining to the ethical issues associated with research on human subjects, informed consent, and the definitional question of whether the intended uses of INDs in the Gulf War constituted research or treatment. The second set consists of immediate policy questions related to the Interim Rule itself; the actual Gulf War experience in the implementation of the rule; alternatives to the Interim Rule, including complete revocation; and the possibility of some form of anticipatory informed consent by service personnel either at recruitment or before deployment.

Finally, a third set of broader, longer-term issues deals with possible conflict (or tension) between the constitutional authority of the President as Commander in Chief and the authority of the Secretary of Health and Human Services under the FDCA, the delegation of that authority to the Commissioner of Food and Drugs under the FDCA, and the interactions between DoD and FDA as they pertain to military drug development and use. This conflict arises from the fact that neither FDCA nor its implementing regulations were developed with

---

[9]Pendergast, who had been FDA Commissioner David Kessler's principal deputy, left FDA for the private sector in early 1998. Moreover, the agency has been without an appointed successor to Kessler since the spring of 1997. In this context, the rule making timetable suggested here may appear optimistic, even unrealistic.

respect to the special needs of military drug development and use. They certainly were not developed for the contingency that arose in the Gulf War, where the DoD concluded it needed to use investigational drugs for prophylactic, non-research purposes. Moreover, although military drug development has been conducted in full compliance with FDA regulations, it has faced difficult problems in adapting to those regulations with respect to prophylactic or therapeutic drugs for defense against CW/BW agents. Finally, it is worth noting that Congress has not enacted clear statutory directives, and the courts have not issued clear interpretations, of how this complex relationship between military drug development and use and the FDA should be organized.

These three sets of issues have both internal and external dimensions for DoD. The internal dimension pertains to those matters over which DoD has control, such as information to military personnel about the risks and benefits of the investigational drugs in question; training of military personnel, both medical and nonmedical, in the administration of IND drug; and record keeping, as well as threat analysis, production, logistics, and the like. These internal matters, however, do influence the debate over the merit of various policies. For example, DoD implementation of the waivers of informed consent for PB and BT was not well-executed in the Gulf War and, consequently, has reflected badly on the policy itself. (See the discussion in Chapter Four, especially regarding Questions A-8c, 8d, 8e, 8f, and 8g.)

The external dimension lies in the reality that policy regarding the potential combat use of investigational drugs does not currently lie within DoD authority but requires the participation and concurrence of FDA and DHHS in both the legal framework governing use and the actual use of drugs within that framework.

THE TEXT OF THE INTERIM RULE

The following is the text of the Interim Rule of December 21, 1990:

> Section 50.23 [21 CFR Part 50], "Exception from general requirements," is amended by adding new paragraph (d) to read as follows:
>
> (d)(1) The commissioner may also determine that obtaining informed consent is not feasible when the Assistant Secretary of Defense (Health Affairs) requests such a determination in connection with the use of an investigational drugs (including an antibiotic or biological product) in a specific protocol under an investigational new drug application (IND) sponsored by the Department of Defense (DOD). DOD's request for a determination that obtaining informed consent from military personnel is not feasible must be limited to a specific military operation involving combat or the immediate threat of combat. The request must also include a written justification supporting the conclusions of

the physician(s) responsible for the medical care of the military personnel involved and the investigator(s) identified in the IND that a military combat exigency exists because of special military combat (actual or threatened) circumstances in which, in order to facilitate the accomplishment of the military mission, preservation of the health of the individual and the safety of other personnel require that a particular treatment be provided to a specified group of military personnel, without regard to what might be any individual's personal preference for no treatment or for some alternative treatment. The written request must also include a statement that a duly constituted institutional review board has reviewed and approved the use of the investigational drug without informed consent. The Commissioner may find that informed consent is not feasible only when withholding treatment would be contrary to the best interests of military personnel and there is no available satisfactory alternative therapy. (2) In reaching a determination under paragraph (d)(1) of this section that obtaining informed consent is not feasible and withholding treatment would be contrary to the best interests of military personnel, the Commissioner will review the request submitted under paragraph (d)(1) of this section and take into account all pertinent factors, including, but not limited to: (i) The extent and strength of the evidence of the safety and effectiveness of the investigational drug for the intended use; (ii) The context in which the drug will be administered, e.g., whether it is intended for use in a battlefield or hospital setting or whether it will be self-administered or will be administered by a health professional; (iii) The nature of the disease or condition for which the preventive or therapeutic treatment is intended; and (iv) The nature of the information to be provided to the recipients of the drug concerning the potential benefits and risks of taking or not taking the drug. (3) The Commissioner may request a recommendation from appropriate experts before reaching a determination on a request submitted under paragraph (d)(1) of this section. (4) A determination by the Commissioner that obtaining informed consent is not feasible and withholding treatment would be contrary to the best interests of military personnel will expire at the end of 1 year, unless renewed at DOD's request, or when DOD informs the Commissioner that the specific military operation creating the need for the use of the investigational drug has ended, whichever is earlier. The Commissioner may also revoke this determination based on changed circumstances.

James S. Benson

Deputy Commissioner of Food and Drugs

Friday, December 21, 1990

Louis W. Sullivan

Secretary of Health and Human Services

Chapter Two

THE HISTORY OF THE INTERIM RULE

The history of the Interim Rule involves the discussions that led to its promulgation; the immediate, but limited, controversy surrounding it; and the FDA decision seven years after the Gulf War to complete the rule-making process. The brief text of the Interim Rule was provided at the end of Chapter One. Its main provisions are these: A process is established by which a determination may be made by the Commissioner of Food and Drugs, pursuant to a written request by the Assistant Secretary of Defense (Health Affairs) (ASD[HA]), that obtaining informed consent for the use of investigational drugs is "not feasible" for a "specific military operation involving combat or the immediate threat of combat." The request must indicate that a duly constituted IRB has reviewed and approved the use of the IND without informed consent. The commissioner, in reaching his or her decision, may find that obtaining informed consent is not feasible "only when withholding treatment would be contrary to the best interests of the military personnel" and when "no available satisfactory alternative therapy" is available.

THE MEMORANDUM OF UNDERSTANDING BETWEEN DOD AND FDA

A Memorandum of Understanding (MOU) has existed between DoD and FDA for some time that pertains to the "investigational use of drugs, antibiotics, biologics, and medical devices" by DoD (52 FR 33472, September 3, 1987).[1] It provides that clinical testing of investigational drugs, biologics, or medical devices under programs sponsored by DoD, whether conducted within DoD facilities or by a contractor or grantee, will follow FDA regulations governing

---

[1] Initially executed by the Department of Health, Education, and Welfare and DoD in 1964, the MOU was revised in 1974 to indicate the procedures that would be followed "to ensure that the requirements of the Federal Food, Drug, and Cosmetic Act and its implementing regulations are fully met without jeopardizing or impeding the requirements of national security." It was revised again in 1987, and it is this version that is currently in force.

"the investigational use of new drugs [including antibiotics and biologics] and medical devices in human beings" and, further, that such clinical testing will adhere to FDA's informed consent and IRB regulations.

The MOU also states that FDA and DoD "will continue to cooperate in meeting the requirements of the Federal Food, Drug, and Cosmetic Act and its implementing regulations without jeopardizing the mission of the DoD." This involves agreement that FDA will expeditiously review special DoD requirements to meet national defense considerations, including review of available data on a drug, biologic, or device under IND or investigational device exemption (IDE) to determine whether stockpiling for future use or use in an expanded military population is appropriate.

Finally, the MOU addresses circumstances when DoD might find it necessary, "for reasons of national security," to establish security classification for the clinical testing of a drug, biologic, or medical device. Although the general policy of DoD is not to classify medical research and development, classification, if necessary, is solely a DoD determination. If classified studies are required, DoD will submit classified INDs or IDEs, as appropriate, to FDA officers having the required clearances, and FDA will be responsible for maintaining "an appropriate cadre of personnel" with such clearances.

The 1987 MOU summarized the experience under this agreement as indicating

> that the DoD and FDA have a record of cooperation; that human subject concerns have been adequately addressed in DoD-sponsored studies; that the DoD has been able to carry out effectively its responsibilities for national security without compromising the intent of the above-cited statutes and regulations; and that certain exemptions, relieving the DoD from the need to meet the ordinary requirements of the Investigational New Drug (IND) and Investigational Device Exemption (IDE) regulations are no longer necessary.

We discuss the MOU mainly because it did *not* provide a policy framework for dealing with use of investigational drugs for CW/BW defense in the Gulf War. Its scope is restricted to DoD clinical testing of investigational new drugs (including biologics) and devices under basically peacetime circumstances. It states as DoD official policy that military research related to drug, vaccine, and medical device development will be conducted under the same rules as civilian research with respect to the protection of human subjects. But the MOU refers to potential *national security responsibilities* related to the use of INDs only in very general terms and is *silent* on any contingencies that may arise related to CW/BW defense. Thus, as we will discuss later in this report, the MOU may deserve to be revisited in light of the Gulf War.

CAREFUL DELIBERATIONS: 1990

In its *Interim Report* of early 1996, the PAC on Gulf War Veterans' Illnesses observed that DoD and FDA had

> deliberated carefully before enabling, through rule making, DoD to take pyri-
> dostigmine bromide (PB) and botulinum toxoid (BT) vaccine as pretreatments
> for possible CBW agents without FDA approval of the products for that purpose.
> (PAC, 1996b, Executive Summary.)

The agencies, the PAC stated, had undertaken "an urgent and orderly course of action under the circumstances to devise a means to address the real threat of chemical and biological warfare in the Gulf War." (p. 23) The importance of a publicly open process of deliberation cannot be overemphasized, especially since some critics of the Interim Rule have argued that it violates the Nuremberg Code. (*JAMA*, 1996.) The Nuremberg Code was adopted at the end of World War II in response to the outrageous wartime Nazi experiments on concentration camp prisoners, which were conducted in the secrecy of the German war machine.

DoD-FDA Discussions

Following the Iraqi attack on Kuwait, the DoD military medical establishment quickly concluded that the investigational drugs of PB and BT vaccine would possibly be needed for defense against CW/BW agents. Dr. Enrique Mendez, ASD(HA), also decided that DoD would seek FDA approval for its actions and would not take actions with which FDA was not in concurrence. DoD could have reached a different decision. It might have argued that neither the FDCA nor its implementing regulations were written with military drug development and use in mind but were developed to regulate the interstate commerce of commercial drug development and use. It certainly could have argued that the defense against CW/BW threats was never considered in the development of FDCA and its regulations and that no clear congressional statute or judicial guidance existed for such a contingency. Thus, it might have concluded that, under the circumstances, it should issue its own regulations appropriate to the military situation without reference to the FDCA.

That DoD did not do so may be attributable to the urgency of the moment, to its desire to have the decision to use INDs ratified by a civilian agency of government, and to the reluctance of FDA to sanction such action formally. In any event, the decision that was reached had the effect of framing the discussion in terms of FDA regulations, the adequacy of those regulations for dealing with the Iraqi threat, and the DoD's perceived need for an exemption on the issue of informed consent.

We focus here on the discussions between DoD and FDA. Although there were a number of meetings between DoD and FDA, two such meetings indicate both the complexity of the issues and that they were clearly understood early in the discussions. An August 30 meeting reviewed the issues associated with the unusual military medical needs of ODS, especially possible deployment of IND status medical products (Lehman, 1990).[2]

The major issue discussed dealt with the DoD request for waiver of the requirement of informed consent. DoD had reviewed the detailed Code of Federal Regulations (CFR) requirements for use of investigational drugs and had concluded that the requirement for informed consent (21 CFR 50) could not be met "in armed conflict and in circumstances of potential armed conflict for deployed and deployable units." It requested immediate relief from this requirement, either by waiver or by a new regulation.

FDA regulates drugs (including biologics) and medical devices (a) produced in the United States and shipped in interstate commerce for use in this country; (b) produced in the United States and exported for overseas distribution and use; and (c) produced overseas and imported to the United States. The first (a) must comply with all regulations governing INDs in the investigational stage and must meet the criteria of safety and effectiveness for approval of an NDA. The last (c) must meet the safety and effectiveness criteria for NDA approval. Drugs and devices produced overseas for distribution to and use in other countries do not fall under authority of the U.S. FDA.

In this context, FDA responded to DoD at the time with two main possible courses of action. First, for IND products exported from the United States and used overseas, the export licensing requirement (21 CFR 312.110), under which informed consent and investigational labeling are not required, was deemed "the quickest and most feasible approach." In such cases, FDA would review each product for safety and, under the MOU, would review available data to determine the appropriateness of use in an expanded military population.[3]

Second, for investigational products used in the United States, for example, to vaccinate troops before overseas deployment, an amendment to the regulations

---

[2]FDA participants included Dr. Stuart Nightingale, Associate Commissioner for Health Affairs (HA); Mr. Duncan, Deputy Associate Commissioner (HA); Margaret Porter, Chief Counsel (OGC); Ms. Witt (OGC); Ms. Wion (OGC); Mr. Geyer (OGC); Dr. Carl Peck, Director, Center for Drug Evaluation and Research (CDER); Dr. James Bilstad, Director, Office of Drug Evaluation II (CDER); Dr. Botstein, Deputy Director, Office of Drug Evaluation I (CDER); Dr. Elaine Esber, Deputy Director, Center for Biologics Evaluation and Research (CBER); Mr. Hoeting, Office of Compliance; and others. DoD participants included Dr. Ronald Clawson, Lt. Col. Lehmann, Lt. Col. Berezuk, Dr. Brandt, and Mr. Winchester.

[3]The autoinjectors for administering diazepam to treat seizures for individuals exposed to PB actually constituted a third possibility, since they were produced overseas and shipped directly to the ODS theater of operations.

(21 CFR 50) signed by the Secretary of Health and Human Services (HHS) would be necessary. This might require Office of Management and Budget (OMB) clearance and could take weeks. Time would not permit the publication of an NPRM. Therefore, a public announcement before completion of such an amendment was thought to be necessary. Drafting of an amendment was under way at FDA. Both options were considered necessary, on the assumption that IND products would need to be used both in the United States and in the theater of operations. FDA also made clear that reviews of investigational products would proceed on a case-by-case basis. FDA raised the question of who would resolve "the impasse if FDA decides that it is inappropriate to deploy a particular investigational product that Defense wants to deploy," which was not resolved at this meeting. We address this important policy issue toward the end of this report.

Although the informed consent issue was the primary concern, much discussion focused on the detailed requirements regarding INDs and their use. Those not familiar with FDA and its regulations may find it difficult to appreciate the level of detail that is involved. But we summarize the minutes of this August 30 meeting to convey a sense for precisely this aspect of the issue. Moreover, this detail is important because the actual difficulty DoD had in the Gulf War in complying with these requirements became a focus of the later attack on the merit of the Interim Rule itself. The following topics, derived directly from the Code of Federal Regulations, were considered:

- **Labeling:** FDA regulations require that an IND be labeled "*Caution: New Drug—Limited by Federal (or United States) Law to Investigational Use.*" For investigational items carried by service members, as distinct from those administered by medical personnel, DoD argued that this language could undermine a soldier's confidence in the treatment or even encourage its nonuse. The compromise language discussed was "*FOR MILITARY USE AND EVALUATION ONLY.*" Waiver under existing regulations was thought possible.

- **Promotion and charging for INDs:** This pertained only to commercialization, which would not occur in ODS.

- **Safety reports:** DoD could not report adverse experiences within three working days of a reported event, or submit a written report within 10 days, during armed conflict or in circumstances of potential armed conflict. Filing IND safety reports as expeditiously as possible was acceptable; relaxing civilian requirements did not require a waiver.

- **Annual reports:** DoD could file such reports.

- **General requirements for IND use in clinical investigations:** DoD, as indicated above, concluded that the requirement for informed consent could not be met "in armed conflict and . . . potential armed conflict." It asked for immediate relief from this requirement by waiver or by a new regulation. DoD indicated that it could comply with the requirement for an IRB review.

- **General responsibilities of sponsors:** Commercial sponsors had no reason to deny DoD permission to cross-reference an IND; therefore, DoD IND sponsorship could be granted.

- **Selecting investigators and monitors:** "The concept of an investigator, and investigator responsibilities in these [active conflict] circumstances," the minutes stated, was "incompatible with the operational realities of applied military medicine." DoD requested relief. FDA urged DoD to do the best it could on inventory control in combat. No waiver or revision of the regulation was required.

- **Informing investigators:** DoD was not clear that it could comply with the requirement for an investigator brochure in actual or potential combat, since there might not be an investigator or one might not be present when the investigational product was used, and requested relief. Information on safety and use of investigational medical products would be provided, the minutes record, "to medical and paramedical personnel, and to individual service members for . . . products intended for self-administration." FDA agreed that this requirement could be met by provision of information in any form—technical reports, field manuals, updated information—and that a waiver was not required.

- **Record keeping and record retention:** DoD indicated that it could not comply in conflict situations with the requirements to "record the name of the investigator to whom the drug is shipped, and the date, quantity, and batch or code mark of each shipment." It could and would record the total amount of investigational product used and would retain records in accord with standard military regulations, but relief from FDA requirements was requested.

- **Disposition of unused supply of an investigational drug:** DoD claimed that it could not ensure the return of all unused supplies of an investigational product. "Given the chaotic nature of armed conflict," it requested relief.

- **General responsibilities of investigators:** Given that the concept of an investigator may not be feasible in actual or potential armed conflict, DoD could not comply with the requirements that the investigator conduct the investigation according to a signed investigator statement or plan or obtain informed consent from those to whom investigational medical products would be administered. Relief was requested. An investigational plan acceptable to DoD, i.e., a retrospective survey, should be submitted with the IND. Informed consent should be addressed separately.

- **Control of the investigational drug:** Relief from this requirement was requested on the grounds that investigators might not be able to supervise the self-administration of an investigational product directly.

- **Investigator record keeping and record retention:** Actual or potential conflict limited the ability of DoD to comply with requirements for recording disposition of the drug and case histories and for retaining records, since an on-scene investigator might not be possible. Relief was requested. DoD and FDA agreed that some level of hospital record keeping could be accomplished and waiver of the regulations was not required.

- **Investigator reports:** Although having an investigator may not be feasible in actual or potential armed conflict, DoD would "attempt to collect and provide information on safety and efficacy" of IND products; retrospective data collection was likely to be most feasible. Relief was requested. Waiver was not required.

- **Assurance of IRB review:** DoD agreed to obtain IRB review and approval and report to the IRB all changes in information collection and all unanticipated problems.

- **Inspection of investigator's records and reports:** FDA insisted on having access to all sponsor and DoD records, regardless of whether or not an investigator was involved. FDA access to classified information would require security clearance.

- **Handling of controlled substances:** Controlled substances would be handled according to existing DoD regulations for substances subject to the Controlled Substances Act. Relief from FDA requirements was requested.

The minutes of the September 14 meeting addressed four legal issues related to the use of INDs in support of ODS[4]: (1) whether Title 10 USC 980 prohibited the use of investigational products if informed consent was not obtained; (2) whether FDA's "treatment IND" regulations might provide the authority DoD needed; (3) the process for establishing the authority of the FDA Commissioner to determine that informed consent was "not feasible" in certain military situations; and (4), if such authority was established, DoD's responsibilities under the pertinent regulations. (Sisson, 1990.)

The most important issue was whether the contemplated DoD use of INDs in support of ODS was *research* or *treatment* and whether IND use for treatment was precluded by Title 10 USC 980. "The key legal issue," a memorandum by

---

[4]DoD participants included ADM (Dr.) Edward Martin, Health Affairs; John Casciotti, Office of General Counsel; and LTC George H. Sisson, Command Judge Advocate. FDA participants included Dr. Stuart Nightingale, Associate Commissioner, Health Affairs; Margaret Porter, Chief Counsel; and Dr. Carl Peck, Director, CDER.

the Assistant General Counsel of DoD read, "is whether the potential uses contemplated constitute 'research involving a human being as an experimental subject' within the meaning of this provision." In DoD's judgment, "the potential drug uses are not human subjects research." (Gilliat, 1990.)

Title 10 USC 980 had been added to a DoD appropriations bill in 1972, and its language expressly precluded DoD from using appropriated funds "for research involving a human being as an experimental subject" unless one of two conditions had been met: Either the informed consent of the subject had been obtained in advance; or, for research intended to benefit the subject, the informed consent of the subject *or a legal representative of the subject*" [emphasis added] had been obtained in advance. Therefore, if the contemplated use was for research, informed consent would be required.

How did DoD justify its proposed use of INDs as treatment? The drugs and biologics under consideration for use in ODS, the Gilliat memo argued, were neither "remarkably novel nor experimental in a scientific or medical sense." Some had been subjected to "extensive research" and some had been approved for uses that were not substantially different from the potential military need confronted in ODS. That need was for defense against "the potential unprecedented use of chemical and biological products" in the Gulf. The proposed use of these INDs could include the administration of one or more of them to "very large numbers of U.S. forces" as pretreatment for threatened CW/BW attack. Given the circumstances, the memo argued, "it is clear that the proposed uses are not in any usual sense of the word for 'research' purposes, but rather to assure the best possible preventive and therapeutic treatment possible for all contingencies presented." It was also the case that no alternative therapeutics were available.

Notwithstanding this argument, the Gilliat memo continued, a possible "technical legal" question remained about whether such products must be *legally* classified as "research" because FDA had not "fully approved," i.e., licensed, them for general treatment. Lacking such approval, these products were legally classified as INDs under FDCA, thus restricting their use to investigational purposes only.

The Gilliat memo then discussed in some detail the authority of FDA (under 21 CFR 312.34) to permit the use of INDs for *treatment* under certain limited circumstances for individuals not in an approved clinical trial being conducted under a treatment protocol.[5] Although such authority existed, it was tightly restricted: The trials had to have progressed through certain stages; the drug

---

[5]This authority allows the "off label" use by a physician of a drug approved for one indication for a nonapproved indication.

had to be needed to treat "serious or immediately life-threatening disease"; and it was essential that no satisfactory alternative treatment was available. Where investigational drugs were used under a treatment IND, it was recognized that the primary purpose was treatment; obtaining additional data on safety and effectiveness was clearly secondary. Such authority had been used to approve the use of drugs for patients with HIV disease, for example, while clinical trials continued and while the drugs in question were still investigational. Although use of treatment IND authority required informed consent of subjects under the provisions of 21 CFR 50, this requirement could be waived if obtaining consent was "not feasible."

The memo summarized the DoD position regarding the potential application of the treatment IND regulations in this way:

> In connection with the potential need in Operation Desert Shield for certain treatment uses of the several drugs classified as INDs, it is clear that very unusual circumstances are present. The drugs have all progressed through FDA's IND process sufficiently to establish a high level of confidence on the part of the DOD medical community; the potential effects of the chemical and bio-logical weapons widely reported as available to the Iraqi military are deadly; and the proposed uses, if approved by the FDA, will reflect the best scientific and medical judgment of the U.S. Government. (Gilliat, 1990.)

Returning to 10 USC 980 on the question of whether the proposed ODS uses constituted "research involving a human being as an experimental subject," the memo argued that "the proposed uses of the drugs in question are, in fact, pri-marily treatment uses, not uses primarily for investigational or research pur-poses." It was appropriate to give legal recognition to this distinction in light of the basic purposes of 10 USC 980, which were narrowly restricted to clear research efforts, and given the necessity to assure DoD's ability "to provide to the forces involved in Operation Desert Shield the best preventive and thera-peutic treatment available."

Moreover, this distinction had previously been established in a 1983 DoD Directive on "Protection of Human Subjects in DoD-Supported Research," which defined research as "a systematic investigation . . . designed to develop or contribute to generalizable knowledge." (DoD, 1983.) That directive had authorized the secretaries of the military departments to determine that "unique military requirements dictate the use of drugs or devices not officially approved by the FDA." DoD had an established interpretation that some drugs and devices FDA deemed "investigational" were not considered as "research" under 10 USC 980.[6]

---

[6]One reviewer (Richard A. Merrill) of the draft version of this report wrote:

The legislative history of 10 USC 980 also made clear that Congress, in enacting the provision, "did not have in mind the potential military need for very large scale preventive and therapeutic treatment to deal with battlefield chemical or biological weapon attacks." Rather, the memo argued, referring to the remarks of Sen. Edward Kennedy on the Senate floor in 1972, that Congress was attempting to remedy evils related to clinical research projects, not problems associated with protection of troops in combat situations. The examples cited in 1972 had been the Public Health Service syphilis experiments in Alabama; brain surgery experiments on prisoners to alter their behavior; a test of a birth control pill on women, mostly Mexican-American; withholding of penicillin from patients with strep throat; and whole-body radiation of terminal cancer patients.

Finally, the memo referred again to the precedent in FDA regulations for treatment INDs for distinguishing between use of INDs for research and treatment purposes. The DoD memo had "no trouble concluding that the proposed treatment uses of these drugs—separate from the ongoing clinical trials—are not part of the research program within the meaning of 10 USC §980." Consequently, DoD did not regard 10 USC 980 as

> an obstacle to your [ASD(HA)] efforts to work out with FDA officials appropriate means, including but not necessarily limited to 'treatment use' approvals under FDA regulations, to assure the maximum preparedness of U.S. Forces in Operation Desert Shield.

The FDA response to this argument in the September 14 meeting was to state that it did not wish DoD to proceed under the treatment IND authority of 21 CFR 312.34, but that treatment use should be by "open protocols" under the *regular* provisions of 21 CFR 312. More important, FDA committed itself again to writing a new regulation to determine that informed consent was "not feasible" in certain military situations. However, this regulation still had to be reviewed by the Commissioner of DHHS (including NIH's Office for the Protection of Research Risks), and OMB. DoD would have the opportunity to see and comment on it before it became final. The regulation would give the FDA Commissioner authority to determine on a product-by-product, protocol-by-protocol basis whether to waive the requirement of informed consent for the use of INDs for certain military uses as "not feasible." DoD would then have to request waivers under this authority for each product, explaining why such consent was not feasible. The DoD IRB would have to consider proposed

---

DoD's conclusion that the use of the two agents did not fall under 10 USC §980 seems entirely reasonable [and] should have influenced judgments about whether it was necessary for DoD to comply with or obtain an exemption from the FDA regulations for investigational use. Viewed as an initial matter, particularly given the specificity of the congressional policy reflected in 10 USC §980, one could argue that DoD must comply with the FDA requirements only when it is also obliged to comply with 10 USC §980.

waiver requests before they were sent to FDA. FDA would consider the DoD request and any other relevant factors. It could then grant a waiver of informed consent for a limited time, i.e., for one year or until the end of the military emergency.

The minutes of these meetings, which reflect only some of the discussions between DoD and FDA, make clear that all the issues associated with the subsequent issuance of the Interim Final Rule were identified and the subject of careful deliberation. In support of these deliberations, DoD provided FDA with a list (see Table 1) of IND medical products under consideration for use in Operation Desert Shield. This list shows that, although PB and BT were the primary subjects of discussion, they were not the only investigational products under consideration for use.

DoD Requests Authorization to Waive Informed Consent

The military assessment of the Iraqi CW/BW threat and DoD's discussions with FDA led the U.S. Army Medical Research and Development Command to recommend to the ASD(HA) on October 11, 1990, that DoD seek a waiver of informed consent for the use of PB and BT in ODS. This recommendation became the basis for a letter of October 30, 1990, from Dr. Enrique Mendez, Jr., ASD(HA), to the Assistant Secretary of Health, DHHS. At the request of DoD, this letter was reprinted in its entirety in the preamble to the Interim Rule (55 FR 52814).

The Mendez letter set forth the DoD rationale for seeking authority to waive informed consent for the use of certain INDs in specific military exigencies. It noted that the DoD-FDA MOU recognized that there were "special DOD requirements to meet national defense considerations," and that such requirements were presented by ODS. Contingency planning for ODS had to consider endemic diseases in the Persian Gulf area, a factor whenever troops were deployed overseas, as well as the unusual threats raised by Iraq's "well-publicized capabilities" in CW/BW weapons. Regarding the latter, DoD had determined "that the best preventive or therapeutic treatment calls for the use of products now under 'investigational new drug' protocols of FDA."

These drugs, although not identified by name, were described as "not exotic new drugs," but ones that had "well-established uses," although for contexts different from DoD requirements, and were "believed by medical personnel in both DoD and FDA to be safe." Examples included "a special intramuscular injector" for ready use on the battlefield, a vaccine the CDC have long recognized as the "primary preventive treatment for a particular disease," and a licensed drug in common use at a dosage level higher than the DoD intended to use, although not approved by FDA for DoD's proposed use.

Explicit FDA assistance was sought "on the issue of informed consent." Under the FDCA, Mendez noted, the "general rule" required that any use of an IND, whether for research or treatment, "must be preceded by obtaining informed consent from the patient." The law allowed for exceptions, however, when professionals administering an IND "deem it not feasible" to obtain informed consent. The heart of the DoD argument was the following:

> Our planning for Desert Shield contingencies has convinced us that another circumstance should be recognized in the FDA regulation in which it would be consistent with the statute and ethically appropriate for medical professionals to "deem it not feasible" to obtain informed consent of the patient, that circumstance being the existence of military combat exigencies, coupled with a determination that the use of the product is in the best interests of the individual. By "military combat exigencies," we mean military combat (actual or threatened) circumstances in which the health of the individual, the safety of other personnel and the accomplishment of the military mission require that a particular treatment be provided to a specified group of military personnel, *without regard to what might be any individual's personal preference for no treatment or for some alternative treatment.* [emphasis added]

In all peacetime applications, the letter continued, DoD believed strongly "in informed consent and in its ethical foundations." In such cases, DoD readily agreed to tell military personnel, in accordance with FDA regulations, that research was involved, that risks or discomforts might be experienced, that participation was voluntary, and that refusal to participate carried no penalty. *"But military combat is different"* [emphasis added], Mendez argued, setting forth the doctrine of military authority in the following way:

> If a soldier's life will be endangered by nerve gas, for example, it is not acceptable from a military standpoint to defer to whatever might be the soldiers' personal preference concerning a preventive or therapeutic treatment that might save his life, avoid endangerment of the other personnel in his unit and accomplish the combat mission. Based on unalterable requirements of the military field commander, it is not an option to excuse a non-consenting soldier from the military mission, nor would it be defensible militarily or ethical to send the solider unprotected into danger.

Regarding this last point, the Mendez letter noted that a number of Supreme Court cases had established "that special military exigencies sometimes must supersede normal rights and procedures that apply in the civilian community." Long-standing military regulations made clear that military personnel might be required to submit to medical care judged necessary to "preserve life, alleviate suffering or protect the health of others." However, the nature of military command authority carried special responsibility for the well-being of military personnel. Consequently, the following procedural limitations were proposed for the "not feasible" determination: that waiver decisions be made on a case-by-case basis by the Commissioner of FDA, thus "assuring an objective review outside of military channels"; that written justification be provided for the intended uses of IND drugs and biologics and the specific military circumstances involved; that no satisfactory alternative treatment is available; that available safety and efficacy data support the proposed use of the drug or biologic; that each request be approved by the applicable DoD IRB; and that waivers have time limits.

FDA Rule Making

The Mendez letter set in motion the formal rule preparation processes of FDA, which ended when FDA issued the Interim Rule, "Informed Consent for Human Drugs and Biologics; Determination that Informed Consent is Not Feasible" (55 FR 52814), on December 21, 1990. In a lengthy preamble that included the Mendez letter, FDA explained its rationale for the rule. It acknowledged its responsibility to protect human subjects exposed to IND drugs, "the central role that informed consent plays in ensuring that protection," and that only "the narrowest of exceptions" to this requirement were consistent with FDA responsibilities. However, the agency had concluded that under the special circumstances that might be created by troops in conflict, the agency "may narrowly expand" the authority of the commissioner to determine that obtaining informed consent is "not feasible." It agreed with DoD that obtaining informed consent might not be feasible "in certain combat-related situations" and that withholding IND drugs for treatment would be "contrary to the best interests of military personnel involved."

FDA recognized DoD's "right and responsibility" to make the command decision to send troops into combat and its concomitant responsibility to protect those troops, both individually and collectively. This protection, FDA acknowledged, might include prevention or treatment with an investigational drug. Coming to the heart of its rationale, FDA stated:

> FDA will consider investigational products proposed for military use on a case-by-case basis, and the agency is prepared to waive the requirement of informed consent where it can be documented that use of these agents in combat-related situations serves the best interests of individual soldiers and the military combat units in which they serve. Since these individual soldiers may be required to be exposed to combat, permitting them to choose whether to receive an investigational product that is the only available satisfactory protection against life-threatening conditions, is contrary to their individual best interests and to the welfare of the other soldiers involved. FDA therefore believes that such an exercise of the Commissioner's discretion is ethically justified. (Preamble to the Interim Rule.)

The detailed provisions of the regulation included FDA review of all products for safety and "expanded availability" to a military population. Importantly, the use of IND products would be monitored by DoD and reported to and reviewed by FDA. Since not all combat situations would create the need to waive informed consent, DoD and FDA must determine the justification for a waiver of informed consent for a particular drug, after IRB approval of the use and the waiver, and make a judgment that anticipated use complied with the limited circumstances outlined in the regulation.

DoD and FDA compliance with established ethical principles was addressed explicitly as it bore on the limitations of the rule. The preamble to the Interim Rule read:

> DoD and FDA also emphasize that accepted ethical principles permit waiver of informed consent only where the preventive or treatment is in the best interests of the individuals involved. Therefore, it is not sufficient as an ethical matter to waive informed consent in the military context where obtaining informed consent is "not feasible," unless it is also the case that withholding the treatment would be contrary to the best interests of the individuals involved.

Consequently, the commissioner would waive informed consent only on a product-by-product basis after a finding that there "is no available satisfactory alternative therapy for the intended diagnosis, prevention, or treatment of the disease or condition." The Commissioner would consider the information provided to recipients of the IND drug about potential risks and benefits; known adverse effects; the risks of failing to take the drug in combat situations; whether the disease or condition (i.e., the military threat) was life-threatening, contagious, or highly debilitating; and how the drug was to be administered. Only written DoD requests for waivers would be considered, and these would have to specify a protocol for use of the IND in question, justification for use, and indication of IRB review and approval. Finally, waivers would expire after one year or when DoD informed FDA that the specific military operation creating the need for the investigational drug had ended, whichever was earlier. DoD could then reapply for a waiver if the need continued beyond the year, but this would not preclude the commissioner from revoking or modifying the waiver on the basis of "changed circumstances."

Request for Waivers

One week after issuance of the Interim Rule, DoD wrote two identical letters to FDA Commissioner David A. Kessler, dated December 28, 1990, one regarding PB and the other about pentavalent BT.[7] In these letters, Dr. Mendez asked the commissioner to determine "that obtaining informed consent is not feasible for

---

[7]The PB request was simultaneously filed as an amendment to IND 23,509; the BT request was filed as an amendment to BB-IND 3723.

[these drugs] because of military combat exigencies in Operation Desert Shield." The PB letter read, in part:

> As summarized in enclosure 1 and supported by documentation in the IND file, available evidence supports the safety and effectiveness of pyridostigmine pretreatment, in conjunction with other drugs, for this purpose. If threatened with these chemical weapons, the interests of individual service personnel and the overall needs of the military service will require that pyridostigmine be used by all threatened personnel. No satisfactory alternative regimen involving investigational or approved drug products is available to deal with these life-threatening weapons. Under these circumstances, withholding pyridostigmine from any threatened individual would be contrary to that individual's best interests. The recommendation for use of pyridostigmine without informed consent has been concurred in by a duly constituted institutional review board. (Mendez, 1990b.)

A similar statement was included in the BT letter. (Mendez, 1990a.)

The DoD PB waiver request was reviewed by the Center for Drug Evaluation and Research (CDER). The review group memorandum read, in part:

> The CDER concludes, based on its review of the safety and effectiveness data, that pyridostigmine 30 mg tablets, in conjunction with atropine and pralidoxime, is the only potentially useful pretreatment to reduce mortality after exposure to chemical weapons involving organophosphorous nerve agent. There is no ethical means of carrying out a relevant human efficacy study. In the absence of human data, there is less than full certainty as to pyridostigmine's effectiveness in man at the recommended dose, but the extrapolation from rhesus monkey and other animal data is not unreasonable, and pyridostigmine has been protective to at least some extent in other species studied.

CBER followed a similar process, which resulted in a similar recommendation for BT.

On January 8, 1991, the FDA Informed Consent Waiver Review Group (ICWRG), in a memorandum to the FDA Commissioner (ICWRG, 1991), recommended approval of the DoD-requested waiver of informed consent for use of PB for ODS. The memorandum noted that "pertinent safety data in both animals and humans" existed and that the recommended daily dose of 90 mg (one 30 mg tablet taken every 8 hours, for a total of 90 mg per day) for Gulf War pretreatment was only 10 to 15 percent of the typical daily dosage of 900 mg or greater prescribed for the treatment of myasthenia gravis. However, the review group expressed concern that DoD instructional materials (FM 8-285 and TM 90-4) implied that PB pretreatment use had been proven to be effective in human studies. "Efficacy data are based wholly on studies in animals," the memo stated. DoD then submitted a supplemental information sheet stating that PB had been shown to be effective in animal studies, and FDA concurred with this statement. A similar recommendation was made with respect to BT.

On January 8, 1991, Commissioner Kessler concurred in the recommendations and signed waivers of informed consent for the use of PB for nerve agent pyridostigmine bromide pretreatment and for BT to immunize against botulism, each limited to a 12-month period. One week later, on January 15, the United Nations' deadline for Iraq to withdraw from Kuwait was reached. Withdrawal did not occur, and coalition forces in the Gulf, led by the United States, attacked Iraqi forces. The coalition forces overwhelmed Iraq by massive air assaults, followed by ground attacks. Within six weeks, President Bush ordered a halt to active hostilities. In less than two months, the engagement with the Iraqis was over. In mid-March, Dr. Mendez informed the FDA Commissioner that hostilities had ended and that the waivers were no longer needed.

The Interim Rule became effective immediately on publication. Although "notice and comment" were deemed impracticable under the circumstances, a 30-day public comment period was provided. The comment period resulted in 21 letters to FDA, some of which supported the rule, others of which were highly critical of it. More important was the discussion in the bioethics literature and, to some extent the popular press, followed by litigation in the federal courts.

LITIGATION: 1991

Immediately upon issuance of the Interim Final Rule, a suit was filed in the U.S. District Court for the District of Columbia seeking to enjoin the DoD "from using unapproved drugs on troops taking part in Operation Desert Storm without first obtaining informed consent from the individual military personnel." Plaintiffs were John Doe, an anonymous soldier serving in ODS, and his wife, Mary Doe, also anonymous. They were represented by the Public Citizen Litigation Group of Washington, D.C. Defendants were Louis W. Sullivan, Secretary of Health and Human Services, and Richard Cheney, Secretary of Defense, who responded to the request for injunction with a motion to dismiss. U.S. District Judge Stanley Harris, in a January 31, 1991 opinion, denied the plaintiffs' motion and granted the motion to dismiss, whereupon the plaintiffs appealed to the U.S. Court of Appeals for the District of Columbia. We review these decisions here.

John Doe and Mary Doe v. Louis Sullivan and Richard Cheney, USDC, District of Columbia, 756F. Supp.12, January 31, 1991

In his opinion, Judge Harris summarized the case as follows. The plaintiffs' challenge to the Interim Final Rule (55 FR 52817), codified at 21 CFR 50.23(d)) argued that the regulation violated the FDCA limitations on the use of unapproved drugs on unconsenting humans; that it was a marked departure from long-standing FDA regulations regarding the feasibility of obtaining informed consent; that DoD was planning to exceed the scope of its authority, which prohibited the use of DoD funds for research on involuntary human subjects; and that use of unapproved drugs on military personnel without their informed consent violated their Fifth Amendment right to due process.

Judge Harris held, first, that the plaintiffs' motion was not likely to prevail on its merits; that the decision to use unapproved drugs was "a military decision"; that a long line of cases supported the defendants' claim that courts were ill-equipped to, and therefore should not, intrude on the relationship between enlisted military personnel and their superior officers; and that the Constitution expressly delegated oversight of the armed forces to Congress, which had enacted "comprehensive statutes regulating military life." Regarding the plaintiffs' motion, he wrote:

> It would be difficult to think of a clearer example of the type of governmental action that was intended by the Constitution to be left to the political branches directly responsible—as the Judicial Branch is not—to the electoral process. Moreover, it is difficult to conceive of an area of governmental activity in which courts have less competence. The complex, subtle, and professional decisions as to the composition, training, equipping, and control of a military force are essentially professional military judgments, subject always to civilian control of the Legislative and Executive Branches. The ultimate responsibility for these decisions is appropriately vested in branches of the government which are periodically subject to electoral accountability. (USDC, DC, 756F. Supp. 12, January 31, 1991.)

Judicial interference "in this type of strategic decision," Harris declared, would be improper and, for that reason, dismissed the request for a preliminary injunction.

The judge went on to say that, even if the plaintiffs' claim were subject to judicial review, the Court would deny its motion for preliminary injunction. Two arguments of the plaintiffs involved statutory construction (or meaning): that the regulation violated the FDCA and that DoD was planning to exceed the scope of its statutory authority. The criteria for judging such arguments were that, where the language of a statute was clear, no resort to legislative history was necessary and that, where a statute was silent, courts defer to the agency responsible for its administration. In this case, the statute was silent and the issue turned, therefore, on "whether the agency's answer is based on a permissible construction of the statute."

For DoD, the act in question was the 1985 DoD Appropriations Act, which prohibited the use of DoD funds "for any research involving a human being as an experimental subject" unless that individual's informed consent was first obtained. The plaintiffs argued that the DoD use of unapproved drugs [in ODS] constituted "research," that under FDA regulations DoD must collect data on the efficacy of such drugs, and that any use of unapproved drugs was research per se. Harris held the contrary:

> Plaintiff's definitional argument is not persuasive in light of the DoD Act's plain meaning. The DoD's use of unapproved drugs does not involve the type of scientific investigation under controlled circumstances that "research" connotes. On the contrary, the DoD has responded to very real circumstances and chosen what it views as the best alternative given current knowledge. The primary purpose of administering the drugs is military, not scientific. The fact that the DoD will collect information on the efficacy of the drugs does not transform the strategic decision to use the unapproved drugs in combat into research.

Moreover, he continued, FDA has interpreted the FDCA to permit use of unapproved drugs in a treatment-investigational setting, indicating that Congress did not intend to embrace all uses of such drugs under the term research.

On whether the Interim Final Rule violated the FDCA, the district court also held for the defendants. FDA had adopted §50.23(d) under authority of the statute that allowed exceptions to the informed consent requirement when obtaining such consent was deemed "not feasible" or "contrary to the best interests" of the individuals in question. FDA was not required under the statute to define "not feasible" so narrowly as to mean "impossible," as the plaintiffs argued. In response to the plaintiffs' argument that it was feasible to obtain informed consent in the combat situation for which DoD sought a waiver, Harris stated that FDA's interpretation was entitled to deference unless "arbitrary, capricious, or manifestly contrary to the statute."

On deprivation of due process under the Fifth Amendment, the court held that there were legitimate government interests in preventing unnecessary danger to all troops and in ensuring the accomplishment of the military mission and that these interests were a "counterbalance [to] an individual's interest in being free from experimental treatment without giving informed consent."

Thus the district court concluded that the DoD plan to administer unapproved drugs in ODS and the FDA's interim rule authorizing such use without informed consent constituted "strategic military decisions," and ones that the court declined to second guess. Even if reviewable, however, the court would have dismissed the motion. The plaintiffs' request for injunction was denied and the defendants motion for dismissal was granted.

Doe v. Sullivan, 938 F.2d 1370, No. 91-5019, USApp DC 111, heard March 18, 1991, decided July 16, 1991

The appeal to the U.S. Court of Appeals for the District of Columbia Circuit was argued on March 18, 1991, and decided on July 16. Writing for the court, Judge

Ruth Bader Ginsburg joined by Judge Patricia Wald, held with the plaintiffs that the court had jurisdiction over the issue, but that the government was well within its authority under the law to issue the rule and authorize waivers under the rule. The court did so by a 2-to-1 vote, Judge Clarence Thomas dissenting in support of the government's arguments that the case was moot.

On mootness, even though hostilities had ended with President Bush's declaration on February 17, 1991, the court agreed with the plaintiffs that the controversy was one "capable of repetition, yet evading review." Although the two waivers for PB and BT had been terminated by the time the circuit court heard the case, the rule remained in existence; the government had no intention of withdrawing it; and "interim" rules had often remained in effect for lengthy periods in prior instances. Thus, the case clearly met the "evading review" criterion. On whether it was "capable of repetition," the court held that the likelihood of encountering chemical and biological warfare threats again against U.S. military personnel fell "in the middle ground between cases in which the recurrence prospect is nonexistent or extremely remote, and those in which the probability of repetition is high." The judicial review began when combat was imminent and both the court and Congress, in determining the need, if any, for legislative change subsequent to Desert Storm, "can consider the question Doe tenders most calmly and effectively after the battle fire is extinguished and before it is rekindled."

On the issue of judicial review, the appellate court held that the challenge to Rule 23(d) was "a straightforward one with a commonplace cast," not a "military action" that bars such review. Doe's challenge simply asks "whether the law that governs FDA action permits the measure which that non-military agency has taken." This issue was clearly within the jurisdiction of the court.

On the merits of the plaintiff's petition, however, the appellate court agreed with the district court:

> the FDA's Rule 23(d), we hold, is within that agency's rule-making authority under the governing section of the FDC Act, and is not barred by the 1985 Department of Defense Authorization Act or the due process clause of the Fifth Amendment.

Thus, it upheld the lower court's dismissal of the complaint.

ACTUAL GULF WAR EXPERIENCE WITH PB, BT AND AX

Immediately after the Iraqi invasion, extensive discussions took place within DoD about the use of IND drugs and vaccines for CW/BW defense as the possibility of Iraqi use of CW/BW agents was recognized. A guidance document was issued by United States Army Forces Command (FORSCOM) about the use of nerve agent pyridostigmine bromide pretreatment (IAW FM 8-285, 7 August 1990) soon after ODS began. It addressed, among other things, corps or division command responsibility to decide when "to begin, continue, or discontinue" the NAPP medications based on the threat; the advisory roles of the intelligence officer, the chemical officer, or the surgeon to act in helping the commander make his decision; and the need to reevaluate the combat conditions after three days of self-administration of PB to determine whether or not to continue treatment, emphasizing that orders to continue or discontinue pretreatment "can and should be made at any time, depending on the situation." If PB was to be continued, supplies should be ordered in advance. Continuous administration beyond 21 days was not recommended without a thorough evaluation of the situation. In addition, the document cautioned that unit medical personnel needed to be trained to recognize the signs and symptoms of PB overdose, allergic reactions, and side effects; to give emergency treatment if necessary; to discontinue treatment to alleviate the signs and symptoms of most adverse reactions; and to report to the commander any serious problems with nerve agent pyridostigmine bromide pretreatment administration.

However, during active Gulf War hostilities, which began within days of approval of the PB and BT waivers, the administration of these investigational drugs differed appreciably from expectations based on the DoD policy and the DoD-FDA discussions that led to the Interim Rule. Some U.S. troops received PB tablets, some were vaccinated with botulinum toxoid vaccine (BT), and some were vaccinated against anthrax (AX). In general, record keeping was quite poor.

For PB, a 21-tablet blister pack was dispensed to those service personnel at highest risk of nerve agent exposure. The dosage prescribed was one 30 mg tablet every 8 hours. PB was used by over 250,000 service personnel, but variation in use occurred as a function of unit commander orders. One of the better quality data reports was that of Keeler et al. (1991) on the experience of the XXVIII Airborne Corps. This unit instructed 41,650 solders (6.5 percent women) to take PB at onset of ODS in January 1991. (Keeler et al., 1991.) Individual service members took from one to 21 tablets over periods ranging from 1 to 7 days, with 34,000 soldiers reportedly taking the medication for 6 to 7 days. Reported side effects of PB were experienced by about half the troops, but were considered tolerable; the most common complaints were about side effects that are normal consequences of PB. Intolerance to PB, which was perceived as the need for medical attention, resulted in 483 aid station or clinic visits related to PB. Of these clinic visits, 313 were gastrointestinal; 150 were for frequency or urgency of urination; and there were other manifestations in a few others. As a demonstration of the data problems, the Defense Science Board Task Force on Persian Gulf War Health Effects reported in June 1994 that PB was issued as a nerve agent pretreatment "to nearly all US troops, as well as 45,000 participants from the United Kingdom," (Defense Science Board, 1994, p. 52), a figure later understood to be incorrect.

According to DoD, BT administration was restricted to relatively few units that were thought to be at highest risk; only about 8,000 doses were administered, hardly any to reservists. This vaccine was produced by the Michigan State Department of Public Health.[8]

Information provided to service members and to health care providers was inadequate. Such information was available in training manuals. Information sheets were prepared for both PB and BT. But the actual distribution of information to the troops was highly variable, and postwar testimony by many veterans revealed that the information they received was unsatisfactory, at least in retrospect. This deficiency is perhaps the most telling of all, since authority to waive informed *consent* throws a heavy burden on the obligation to *inform*.

Record keeping was also very poor. This was particularly true for PB, which is self-administered. Without medics to record consumption of medication, there is very little way to overcome this deficiency. In the case of BT, which was administered by medics, record keeping in an individual's yellow shot card was quite uneven. Some record entries were for vaccine A, others for vaccine B, but individuals were not told what they had received. Others were told, and the entries were anthrax vaccine or BT. But there was no uniformity of record keeping during the conflict, which generated substantial criticism afterward.

The disparities between actual events and prior expectations stem from at least four sources. First, time was extraordinarily short. Rule making, which took place in record time, required three months. But only one week was available between the granting of the waivers and actual hostilities. Preparation for orderly processes was next to impossible.

Second, communication flows were quite complicated: They proceeded in the first instance from the ASD(HA) to FDA, then from FDA within DHHS, and from FDA back again to Health Affairs; they then went from Health Affairs to J-4 (Logistics, which includes Medical Readiness) in the Joint Staff; and J-4 was in communication with Central Command (CENTCOM) and BG Robert Belihar, Command Surgeon for CENTCOM during the war. The faithful transmission of complicated information is difficult under normal circumstances. In preparation for active conflict, it is likely to be very, very difficult.

---

[8]The anthrax vaccine, a licensed biologic, was administered to about one-third (150,000) of the troops deployed in the theater. It was also produced by the Michigan State Department of Public Health, and has been extensively used for years by civilian wool factory workers and laboratory workers, and its safety is well documented.

Third, discretion was exercised in the theater of operations that overrode policy that had been agreed upon in Washington. This occurred, for example, in the case of BT administration. Although a waiver of informed consent had been approved for BT, the actual supply of the vaccine that was available for use in the Gulf was limited and inadequate to vaccinate all military personnel. Consequently, informed consent was used as the basis for allocating a scarce resource. As General Belihar later testified,

> We did not have enough vaccine to vaccinate everybody. . . . Now the question is, well, if we have people who are at risk and we don't have enough vaccine to vaccinate everybody, why make it mandatory. So we added the consent factor to it. . . . it seemed reasonable to give them the choice, based upon the fact that you gave the information upon which to base a choice." (PAC meeting, January 12, 1996 transcript.)

In the case of PB, which individual service members self-administered, informed consent was waived. The decision to order troops to take this medication, however, was made by the local unit commander. This occasioned a question at the January 1996 PAC meeting. Ms. Knox, a PAC member, asked General Belihar, "Can you help me understand, too, why the order for PB was a unit command?" Belihar responded:

> I think you cannot, in the moment of battle, coordinate through your component commander up through the CINCCENT [Commander in Chief, U.S. Central Command] to the [Command] surgeon. There are certain things that must be empowered at the unit level.

This response can be understood in two ways, either as an override of FDA-based expectations for some uniformity of the decision to administer PB or, on the other hand, as the exercise of time-honored, and legally protected, exercise of battlefield discretion within the chain of command.

Finally, the administration of these investigational drugs in the Gulf derived from strategic "order of battle" considerations. Again, it is useful to quote General Belihar:

> Well, we had quite a bit of anthrax vaccine, but we did not have nearly enough botulinum toxoid to vaccinate everyone. So we went to the Commander in Chief [Schwarzkopf] and said, "Sir, there's a lot of information that we don't have. We have to go on a best guess. How do we utilize this botulinum toxoid?" I said, "Sir, you've got to make the call because you know the order of battle, I don't." And I will tell you, this whole order of battle is very closely held. I said, "Sir, you make the decision."

He continued a few minutes later with this same theme:

> There was a question that we kept this thing top secret because we wanted to shield the Allies from the fact that we were going to vaccinate. That is not true.

... The reason for the classified nature here is because of the order of battle, because the patterns of vaccine administration would indicate, perhaps, how those troops were going to be employed, and we didn't want to do that.

After the war, PB was implicated as a possible risk factor in Gulf War veterans' illnesses, especially when used in combination with diethyl-m-toluamide (DEET), a pesticide used in the Gulf War by deployed troops. BT and AX were also cited as possible causes for some veterans' illnesses. Most pertinent, however, is the fact that the manner of control and administration of these drugs has been used to call into question the merit of the initial policy embodied in the Interim Rule.

THE PRESIDENTIAL ADVISORY COMMITTEE

The PAC on Gulf War Veterans' Illnesses was established in early 1995 by President Clinton to review factors associated with the causes of Gulf War veterans' illnesses. In the course of its deliberations, it considered the issue of use of investigational drugs and the waiver of informed consent. It did so beginning with a December 1995 staff consultation, not a formal meeting, at the PAC offices. Consequently, no PAC member was present, and no transcript was kept.[9] The meeting, among other things, made clear to many of the participants that DoD had seriously considered its approach to this issue at the time and that the contentious issues were quite complex.

In addition, the PAC meeting on January 12, 1996, in Kansas City, Missouri, heard testimony from a number of witnesses. This meeting, chaired by PAC member Arthur Caplan, received testimony from Brig. Gen. Robert Belihar, Chief Surgeon to GEN Norman Schwarzkopf, theater commander in the Gulf War; David Bales, a physician who had served under Belihar; Edward Martin, then–Deputy Assistant Secretary of Defense for Professional Affairs and Quality Assurance, Health Affairs; Edmund G. Howe, director of programs in medical ethics and Professor of Psychiatry, Uniformed Services University of the Health Sciences; Nightingale, Associate Commissioner for Health Affairs, FDA; and Alta Chara, Professor of Law and Medical Ethics, University of Wisconsin-Madison.

On the bases of these meetings, the PAC, in its *Interim Report* of February 1996, drew three conclusions. First, it noted, as indicated above, that DoD and FDA had

---

[9]Participants included George Annas, Boston University; Edward Martin, Health Affairs; Edmund Howe, the Uniformed Services University of the Health Sciences, DoD; Stuart Nightingale, FDA, Gary Ellis, the Office for the Protection of Human Subjects; his predecessor, Charles McCarthy (who was in that position at the time of the Gulf War); Joan Porter, PAC staff; and others.

deliberated carefully before enabling, through rulemaking, DOD to take pyridostigmine bromide (PB) and botulinum toxoid (BT) vaccine as pretreatment for possible CBW agents without FDA approval of the products for that purpose.

Second, the report criticized FDA for having "failed, in the five years since the Gulf War, to devise better long-term methods governing military use of drugs and vaccines for CBW defense." (PAC, 1996b, Executive Summary.) The text also criticized FDA for not having "been proactive in addressing public comments on the interim final rule." (PAC, 1996b, p. 23.) The PAC further argued that when a waiver of informed consent is granted, "the government has a strong obligation to conduct long-term follow-up of military personnel who receive investigational products." (PAC, 1996b, p. 23.) Third, the PAC "also found DOD's inability to produce records of who received PB or BT indicative of much need for wholesale improvement in the government's performance on medical recordkeeping during military engagements." (Executive Summary). The body of the report extended this criticism to include anthrax vaccine and, rather ruefully, noted that there was "little possibility now of developing reliable data about which or how many persons received these products." (PAC, 1996b, p. 23.) The report also criticized DOD's rationale for keeping vaccination records secret. "This requirement," it stated, "confused and complicated recordkeeping procedures and hindered systematic follow-up of health issues." (PAC, 1996b, p. 23.)

Consequently, the *Interim Report* contained the following two recommendations:

- Given that FDA's Interim Final Rule permitting waiver of informed consent for use of unapproved products in a military exigency is still in effect, DoD should develop enhanced orientation and training procedures to alert all service personnel that they may be required to take drugs or vaccines not fully approved by FDA if a conflict presents serious threat of chemical and biological warfare. (PAC, 1996b, Executive Summary and p. 24.)

- If FDA decides to reissue the Interim Rule as a final rule, it should first issue a NPRM. Among the areas that specifically should be revisited are adequacy of disclosure to service personnel; adequacy of record keeping; long-term follow-up of individuals who receive investigational products; review by an institutional review board outside of DoD; and additional procedures to enhance understanding, oversight, and accountability. (Executive Summary and p. 24.)

In its *Final Report* of December 31, 1996, the PAC evaluated the government's response to its *Interim Report* recommendations. It commended DoD for providing information about tick-borne encephalitis (TBE) to U.S. troops deployed in Bosnia and for obtaining informed consent from those troops to whom the

TBE vaccine was being administered.[10] (PAC, 1996c, p. 20.) However, it also noted that DoD "had made no specific response" to educating troops about the use of investigational pharmaceuticals. Given that the Interim Final Rule remained in effect, the PAC again recommended that DoD

> develop enhanced orientation and training procedures to alert service person-nel they could be required to take investigational drugs or vaccines not fully approved by FDA if a conflict presents a serious threat of exposure to CBW agents. (PAC, 1996c, p. 20.)

The *Final Report* noted that FDA "is now considering the Interim Final Rule in conjunction with guidelines for CBW agent prophylaxis approval," but also expressed concern about the amount of time—nearly six years—that FDA was taking "to move forward with opening up the Interim Final Rule . . . for public comment." (PAC, 1996c, p. 20.)

The PAC *Final Report* had two findings pertaining to the use of investigational drugs. First, it noted that FDA "is moving toward soliciting public comment on *alternatives* [emphasis added] to the Interim Final Rule" but again expressed serious concern about the amount of time that had been taken. (PAC, 1996c, p. 27.) Second, it found that DoD had not been responsive to the recommen-dation that it should routinely inform recruits and troops, through orientation and training, about "the possible use of investigational drugs or vaccines for chemical and biological warfare purposes." This lack of response, the PAC concluded, "contributes to the perception of many that U.S. troops were inap-propriately subjected to investigational drugs or vaccines during the Gulf War." (PAC, 1996c, pp. 27–28.)

The PAC then made the two recommendations. It again recommended that DoD "develop enhanced orientation and training procedures" (p. 52). It also recommended that "FDA should solicit timely public and expert comment on *any rule* [emphasis added] that permits waiver of informed consent for use of investigational products in military exigencies." Among the areas it recom-mended be revisited were the adequacy of disclosure to service personnel; the adequacy of record keeping; long-term follow-up of individuals who receive investigational products; review by an IRB outside of DoD; and additional pro-cedures to enhance understanding, oversight, and accountability. (PAC, 1996c, p. 52.)

The departments of Defense, Health and Human Services, and Veterans Affairs responded to the PAC *Final Report* through the Persian Gulf Veterans' Coordi-nating Board on March 7, 1997 (PGVCB, 1997). FDA concurred with the PAC

---

[10]TBE vaccine is used against an endemic infectious disease, not against a BW agent, and thus its clinical testing does not raise the same questions as do PB and BT.

recommendation. It indicated that it had "carefully evaluated" the PAC recommendations since its *Interim Report,* had discussed the issues with DoD, and noted that the issues raised "are complex and require extensive coordination." FDA was preparing to solicit public comment on whether it should "finalize the Interim Rule, modify it, or eliminate it completely." One part of this process involved exploration of "the approval mechanisms that should be applied to drug and biological products that may be used in military or civilian exigencies." (PGVCB, p. 12.)

The DoD concurred with the PAC recommendation about the need for enhanced orientation and training. It acknowledged that, although medical personnel who participated in ODS were thoroughly briefed about the side effects of PB, this information "did not, in most cases, get down to the individual service member." Some service members' concerns could have been alleviated, DoD responded, "had they known that the side effects they experienced were, in fact, attributed to the known side effects of PB, and which in most cases would go away as the service member became tolerant to those effects of PB." (PGVCB, p. 13.) Consequently, all new and existing stockpiles of PB "will contain appropriate labeling" informing the individual service member of potential side effects and warnings for use.

Regarding orientation and training, DoD responded that it already conducts such programs for new troops "on the chemical and biological threat and on the countermeasures which may be needed." (PGVCB, p. 13.) It acknowledged that "more needs to be and will be done" within the coming year. The stated goal of the DoD is

> that every service member is fully informed during orientation and training of the health risks, benefits, and proper use of all medical countermeasures, and, that when used, such countermeasures are documented and maintained as part of the individual's health record.

Given the potential for CW/BW threats in future conflicts, the DoD sees having a fully informed service member as critical to troop protection. The troop information program and a new DoD medical surveillance policy, DoD asserted, will contribute to enhanced soldier welfare.

Finally, given that the Interim Rule was still in effect, DoD indicated that it would prepare orientation and training procedures

> to alert service personnel [that] they may be required to take drugs or vaccines not fully approved by FDA if a conflict presents a serious threat of chemical and biological warfare. (PGVCB, p. 13.)

The PAC was extended through October 1997, during which time it continued to hold hearings around the country. On July 29, 1997, at a public meeting in

Buffalo, New York, Mary Pendergast, Deputy Commissioner of FDA, announced the agency's intention to complete the rule-making process. Step One of that process was to publish a formal "Request for Comments" in the *Federal Register*. A possible Step Two was to convene a conference focused on issues raised in the comments. The next step would be to issue an NPRM. The final step would be issuance of a final rule.

Chapter Three

WHAT USES OF DRUGS ARE INVESTIGATIONAL?

The immediate policy issues associated with the Interim Rule and its alternatives require us to consider a level of detail that is characteristic of FDA regulation but unfamiliar to many outside the drug evaluation process. Before dealing with those detailed issues, however, we address the question of what *investigational* means.

The critics of the Interim Rule argue that it was a violation of the basic ethical principles governing research on human subjects in its failure to require informed consent for investigational drugs. This argument is politically salient because of the history of abuse of human subjects in medical experiments, a history shared by both military and civilian agencies of the federal government and by nongovernment institutions and investigators. This history is fresh in our thinking, partly because 1997 was the 50th anniversary of the Nazi doctors' trial and the promulgation of the Nuremberg Code (*JAMA*, 1996, 276). Also in 1997, President Clinton publicly apologized to the survivors of the Public Health Service's Tuskegee Syphilis Study. These events had been preceded by the report of the Advisory Committee on Human Radiation Experiments (ACHRE, 1996), a 1993 Institute of Medicine report on the health effects of mustard gas and Lewisite (Pechura and Rall, 1993). This history forcefully reminds us of the need for continued vigilance regarding the ethics of human experimentation. But it should neither blind us to learning from that experience nor relieve us from the obligation to examine the particulars of the Gulf War to assess whether and how they differ from these episodes of abuse.

Did the use of investigational drugs under the Interim Rule in the Gulf War constitute research? A definitional excursion is essential to clarify the policy implications associated with the terms "investigational," "research," and medical "practice" or treatment. The Interim Rule applies to "an investigational drug or biologic," and the two waivers granted under it were for drugs FDA classified as investigational. The pertinent questions in this exercise are the following:

- What does *research* mean and how does it differ from *medical practice*? What is the conceptual basis for distinguishing between the two? How does the experiment-therapy boundary or the *experiment-therapy continuum* help in distinguishing between these activities? How does the Belmont Report (National Commission, 1979) answer these questions?

- What does *investigational* mean, especially when the FDA uses it to classify a therapeutic product, such as a drug, vaccine, or medical device? Does a bright, orange line separate *investigational* from *noninvestigational*? Or does *investigational* identify a gray zone in which several meanings exist?

- What is the relationship between *investigational*, as used by FDA; *research* and *practice*, as used in the Belmont Report; and *research*, as used in 10 USC 980? Does *research* mean the same as *investigational*? Does *investigational* always and exclusively mean *research*, or does it sometimes also include *practice*? Have some "investigational" drugs been studied sufficiently to warrant a judgment by experts that they are safe and effective for treatment use?

- How do the requirements for *informed consent* by human subjects of research intersect with the FDA requirements for the use of investigational drugs?

- Are *exceptions* to the informed consent requirement for research involving human subjects authorized under Title 10 USC 980? Are exceptions to these requirements authorized under FDCA?

At issue is whether FDA classification of a drug as investigational means that its use, for any purpose, automatically and without exception, constitutes "research" and, if so, whether informed consent is required. However, if *investigational* has a range of possible meanings, one of which is a justifiable use for treatment, then the question is whether informed consent may be waived for some treatment uses. The complexity of the definitional task is suggested by the sustained argument over these terms, which requires that we inquire closely into their meanings and lay out the policy implications of the various definitions.

The discussion is complicated by two other factors. First, the point of view adopted by the parties to the debate is strongly influenced by their primary referent. These referents include the Nuremberg Code, the Belmont Report, Sec. 1401(c)(1) of the DoD Authorization Act of 1985, and the statutory provisions and implementing regulations of FDCA. Consequently, the discussion sometimes concerns general principles and at other times specific, legally defined applications. At all times, it requires a struggle to disentangle and analyze terms and meanings. Second, it is often the case that substantial subjectivity, even partisanship, characterizes the definitional discussion, making clear that the task is not simply a scientific exercise but is often about conflicts in underlying values.

THE EXPERIMENT-THERAPY CONTINUUM

The basic concept behind the definition of *investigational* is the research-practice boundary or the experiment-therapy continuum. This continuum, which is usually implicit but needs to be made explicit, embraces both research and practice (see Fox and Swazey, 1974; National Commission, 1979; Sabiston, 1979; Robertson, 1979). It has medical-scientific, regulatory, and informed consent dimensions, which overlap each other without being congruent.

The continuum is conceptually applicable to all medical innovations, including procedures and therapeutic products. In the development of a new medical procedure, or of a new therapeutic product, such as a drug, biologic, or medical device, a progression can be observed, albeit one involving many iterative steps, from laboratory research to clinical investigation, including clinical trials, and then to clinical practice. This is the *medical-scientific* dimension of the continuum.

In the case of drugs, vaccines, and medical devices, there is a *regulatory* overlay. Drugs and biologics are regulated in similar fashion; devices are treated somewhat differently. For drugs, FDA governs the transition from unregulated (preclinical) laboratory research to clinical research involving human subjects by requiring an IND application; it also regulates the transition from the investigational stage to the commercial market by requiring an NDA, which is subjected to extensive FDA review for safety and effectiveness before approval is granted for marketing and which requires postmarketing surveillance after approval. The language of FDCA Sec. 505(a) makes clear the nature of the above controls. It reads:

> No person shall introduce or deliver for introduction into interstate commerce any new drug, unless an approval of an application filed pursuant to subsection (b) or (j) is effective with respect to such drug.

Finally, the *informed consent* overlay governs the protection of human subjects: This overlay includes FDA regulations for drugs (21 CFR 50; 21 CFR 56) and the DHHS rule for NIH and CDC clinical research (45 CFR 46); the latter rule, also known as the Common Rule, has been adopted by all federal government agencies.

These three overlays on the experiment-therapy continuum are not described by a clear set of terms having universal acceptance, unambiguous definitions, and consistent applications. Terms that are roughly comparable are not synonymous. Although the two poles of the continuum—the solely experimental and clearly established therapy—are distinct, the territory between them is a proverbial gray zone; no bright orange line divides activities along the continuum.

The continuum is portrayed graphically in Figure 1, which depicts "research" and "treatment" (at the top and bottom of the figure) as overlapping. We can say the following about this depiction. First, research encompasses preclinical, clinical, and evaluative activities occurring after a medical innovation is introduced to clinical practice. But not all clinical research is therapeutic, i.e., intended for the benefit of the individual research subject. Phase I and Phase II trials may or may not benefit the individual human subject, who is a volunteer, but may be intended solely to generate scientific knowledge of benefit to future patients. However, much clinical research is intended to generate both scientific knowledge and therapeutic benefit to the individual subject of research. Moreover, much therapy clearly lies beyond the research stage. For clinical procedures, however, no clear demarcation of the boundary between research and treatment exists, whereas in the case of drugs, the boundary is defined as an artifact of FDA regulations.

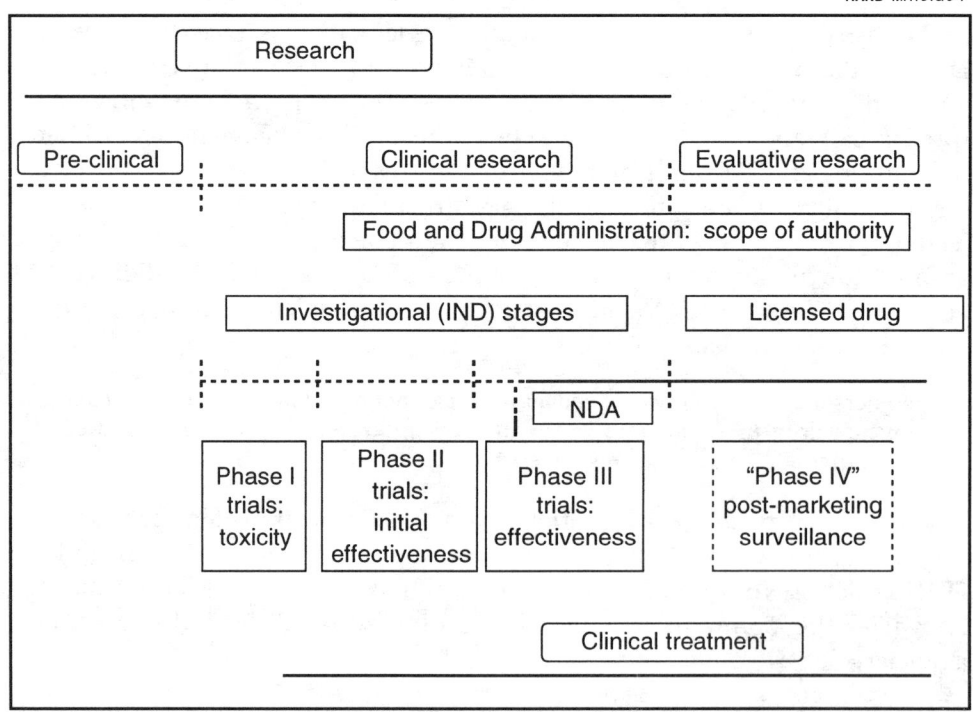

RAND *MR1018/9-1*

Figure 1—Experiment-Therapy Continuum

Second, FDA regulatory authority encompasses all clinical research on therapeutic products under its jurisdiction (drugs, biologics, medical devices)—the "investigational" (or IND) stage; the period after submission of a new drug application (or NDA), during which a drug is evaluated for licensing and introduction to commercial marketing; and postmarketing surveillance (Phase IV studies) after approval. Licensing is based on clinical evidence of safety and effectiveness, but also involves determinations about the adequacy of the manufacturing processes and capabilities, as well as considerations related to labeling.

Third, some research and clinical evaluation continues after a drug or procedure has moved beyond the research stage, has been introduced into clinical practice, and has achieved recognized status as established therapy. This is represented here as "evaluative research" as it applies generally to all medical innovation, the health services research domain of effectiveness and outcomes research, and as "Phase IV" research as it pertains to continuing studies of FDA-approved drugs and vaccines.

THE BELMONT REPORT

The foundation document of the ethical principles governing research on human subjects is the Nuremberg Code, issued at the Nazi doctors' war crimes trials in 1947. The first article of the Code states:

> 1. The voluntary consent of the human subject is absolutely essential.
>
> This means that the person involved should have legal capacity to give consent; should be so situated as to be able to exercise free power of choice, without the intervention of any element of force, fraud, deceit, duress, over-reaching, or other ulterior form of constraint or coercion; and should have sufficient knowledge and comprehension of the elements of the subject matter involved as to enable him to make an understanding and enlightened decision. This latter element requires that before the acceptance of an affirmative decision by the experimental subject there should be made known to him the nature, duration, and purpose of the experiment; the method and means by which it is to be conducted; all inconveniences and hazards reasonably to be expected; and the effects upon his health or person which may possibly come from his participation in the experiment.
>
> The duty and responsibility for ascertaining the quality of the consent rests upon each individual who initiates, directs or engages in the experiment. It is a personal duty and responsibility which may not be delegated to another with impunity. (JAMA, 1996; p. 1691.)

Following the Nuremberg Code, there have been other formulations, such as the Helsinki Declaration and, most important for the United States, the Belmont Report. The Belmont Report was the product of the National Commission for the Protection of Human Subjects of Biomedical and Behavioral Research (1979). The commission was created in 1974, following public revelations in the prior two years about the Public Health Service Tuskegee Syphilis Study, abuses involving unapproved medical experiments, coerced sterilizations, psychosurgery, and research involving prisoners (see Schuchardt, 1994).

The commission was charged by the National Research Act of 1974 "to identify the basic ethical principles that should underlie the conduct of biomedical and behavioral research involving human subjects" and to develop guidelines to ensure that these principles were adhered to in such research. The report identified three basic ethical principles—respect for individuals, beneficence, and justice—that should underlie the conduct of biomedical and behavioral research involving human subjects:

- *Respect for individuals in the conduct of research involving human subjects* encompasses two ethical convictions: first, that persons should be treated as autonomous agents; and second, the persons with diminished autonomy are entitled to protection.

- *Beneficence* involves attempting to ensure that the human subjects involved in research benefit from it.

- *Justice* involves the questions of who should benefit from research and who should bear its burdens.

The report then articulated three applications of these principles—informed consent, risk-benefit evaluation, and selection of subjects:

- *Informed consent* to participation in research involves three aspects: the provision of information to the research subjects, understanding or comprehension by the recipient of the information, and voluntary choice to participate.

- *Risk-benefit calculus* requires the careful analysis of a particular intervention and the provision of information to the subject about the nature and scope of the risks and benefits.

- *Selection of subjects* requires that no individual or group of individuals be unfairly selected to bear the burden of experimentation or be unfairly excluded from sharing the benefits.

To develop guidelines for the protection of research subjects, the commission had to distinguish between research and established medical practice. It acknowledged that the distinction was "blurred," partly because these activities often occur simultaneously. The key paragraph of the Belmont Report reads as follows:

For the most part, the term "practice" refers to interventions that are designed solely to enhance the well-being of an individual patient or client and that have a reasonable expectation of success. The purpose of medical or behavioral practice is to provide diagnosis, preventive treatment or therapy to particular individuals. By contrast, the term "research" designates an activity designed to test an hypothesis, permit conclusions to be drawn, and thereby to develop or contribute to generalizable knowledge (expressed, for example in theories, principles, and statements of relationships). Research is usually described in a formal protocol that sets forth an objective and a set of procedures designed to reach that objective.

However, the commission did state a general rule that, in situations where research and treatment are carried on together, "if there is any element of research in an activity, that activity should undergo review for the protection of human subjects."

Two appendixes in the report wrestled with the research-treatment distinction. Sabiston addressed the "boundaries between biomedical research involving human subjects and the accepted or routine practice of medicine," with an emphasis on surgery. "As one pursues this subject [of boundaries]," he wrote, "it becomes evident that *there is no dividing line which can be consistently agreed upon by any group of authorities on the subject*" [emphasis added]. In Sabiston's view, "such an arbitrary division [between medical practice and research] is simply impossible, at least if determined on a rational basis." Although medical practice that was "established beyond reasonable doubt" and research that was "clearly experimental" were easily distinguished, Sabiston found "a definite 'gray zone' in which practice and research overlapped and objective classification was extraordinarily difficult."

Robertson addressed the legal implications of physician activities "that occur on the boundary between research and the accepted practice of medicine." He uses "on the boundary" and "boundary activity" synonymously with "innovative therapy," characterizing the latter as activity that subjects patients "under the guise of therapy to risky, untested procedures without the safeguards that apply to experimentation." Although the phrase "on the boundary" implies a clear demarcation between research and accepted practice *within* the context of protocol-based research, Robertson was actually using this term, and that of innovative therapy, to describe that which is *neither* protocol-based research *nor* established therapy, but activity that appears to be "on the edge" of these activities. This usage is reasonable given that the commission was concerned about procedures that departed "in a significant way" from standard practice but that were not conducted according to a research protocol. Such procedures were *experimental* in that they constituted both a potential and real source of abuse of human subjects. Hence Robertson's discussion is not pertinent to the current discussion.

Parenthetically, it is important to note that no attention was given in the Belmont Report to FDA or its regulations for drug development. The report made no mention of the fact that, under FDCA regulations, radically experimental drugs or vaccines could not be used for research or treatment without a rigorous, FDA-approved protocol. The problems the Belmont Report addressed did not lie in this direction. The report certainly did not address the hypothetical, which became real in the Gulf War, in which a product, such as PB, licensed by FDA as safe and effective for one indication but in a late "investigational" stage for a different indication, was proposed for use as "treatment" (or pre-treatment) in military combat. Neither did it address the BT situation, where an IND vaccine routinely used for protective purposes for at-risk individuals was being proposed for similar DoD use. Thus, although the report provides the conceptual framework for bioethicists in their reasoning about the issues under discussion, that framework is not sufficiently developed to embrace these issues from the perspective of drug development and use.

ETHICAL CONSIDERATIONS

Understandably, a regulation that authorized the waiver of informed consent for the use of investigational drugs under some military circumstances generated substantial discussion about the ethical issues associated with its use. Discussion included both justification and criticism.

An early ethical defense of the interim rule appeared in the *Hastings Center Report.* Howe and Martin (1991),[1] briefly reviewed the CW/BW threat posed by Iraq, the "compounds" (referring in general to drugs and vaccines and, in particular, to PB and BT) available for protecting service personnel from these threats, the investigational status of these compounds under FDCA, and their scientific and clinical status.

They then posed two ethical questions:

> Should service persons be given these [investigational] compounds? and, if the answer was yes, Should servicepersons be given the opportunity to grant or withhold their consent, as they would if they were research subjects?

Extensive review of the data by DoD, FDA, and HHS had resulted in a decision to give the compounds to service members, to inform them of the compounds' investigational status, including side effects and risks, but not to obtain their informed consent.

---

[1] Howe was associate professor of psychiatry and director of programs in medical ethics, Department of Psychiatry, Uniformed Services University of the Health Sciences. Martin, a physician and career Public Health Service officer, was then Deputy Assistant Secretary of Defense for Professional Affairs and Quality Assurance, Health Affairs.

A major justification put forward by Howe and Martin for this decision was that the use of these compounds was for "preventive or therapeutic treatment as opposed to research." They found support for this distinction in the Belmont Report and the Declaration of Helsinki (World Medical Association, 1997). The former states that treatment usually involves interventions intended solely for the benefit of a particular individual. The fact that "some forms of practice" provide benefits, to others, i.e., knowledge of a general nature, "should not confuse the general distinction between research and practice." The Helsinki Declaration distinguished between medical research whose purpose was "essentially diagnostic or therapeutic for a [given] patient" and that which was intended to be "purely scientific and without direct diagnostic or therapeutic value" to those subjected to it.

Howe and Martin also noted that, although the Nuremberg Code was explicit about the "absolutely essential" requirement of voluntary consent to human experimentation, it was silent regarding clinical research. Using the compounds in question without informed consent, they argued, was consistent with the spirit, if not the letter, of other parts of the Nuremberg Code regarding the conduct of experiments to avoid "unnecessary physical and mental suffering" and to protect against "even remote possibilities of injury, disability, or death."

But since the primary purpose of the use of these compounds in the Gulf War was not research, "the degree, if any, to which their use should be construed as experimental, even according to the two codes that address therapeutic research [Belmont, Helsinki] is open to question." Nevertheless, because these compounds were classified as INDs under the FDCA and "because some generalizable data will be collected concerning the effect of using these compounds," the authors acknowledged "a small research dimension" associated with their use.

The compounds were considered investigational, Howe and Martin argued, for two reasons: first, "they had not been studied to the extent normally required for drugs' commercial use;" and second, because exposing human subjects to the chemical and biological agents that the compounds were intended to protect against would be unethical. However, given that the safety and protective effectiveness of these compounds might differ, "the ethical justification for using each compound before or during combat must be separately determined" (i.e., on a case-by-case basis). It was necessary, therefore, that, in addition to DoD review, experts outside the DoD review both the scientific merits and ethical bases underlying DoD's proposed use of these compounds. Thus, FDA and DHHS conducted external review of these compounds. The conclusion of all parties was that the potential benefits of use were "substantial" and the risks of harm were "extremely small."

The ethical issue then turned on whether service personnel "should have the option of giving or withholding informed consent." The authors then elaborated on military research ethics. No differences between military and civilian research subjects were justified in peacetime. However, "the ethical context shifts," when investigational compounds are used for service personnel in combat or combat-ready situations:

> The principle of preventing unnecessary harm to servicepersons (and enhancing the mission by protecting all servicepersons) *overrides all other values* [emphasis added]; and the principle of respect for persons is fulfilled by maintaining the military's explicit and implicit promise to servicepersons to protect them from unnecessary harm. (Howe and Martin, 1991, p. 22.)

Respect for persons, which differs from allowing individuals to grant or withhold consent, is thus predicated on the military keeping its promise to protect individuals. It is also accomplished, insofar as possible, by fully informing service members about the investigational compounds they will be taking:

> They [service personnel] should be informed that these [compounds] have not been tested vigorously under battlefield conditions; they should be told of the risks and expected benefits so far as they can be identified; they should be warned that the expected benefits do not include prevention of all harms from chemical or biological attack; and they should be made familiar with known side effects of the compounds. (Howe and Martin, 1991, p. 22.)

These shifts from the ethical principles that apply in civilian situations result from the unique obligations of service personnel to their country and to those with whom they serve. Service personnel "are willing to sacrifice their lives if necessary to benefit fellow servicepersons or to further the military's mission." A service member "freely agrees when joining the military to relinquish autonomy" to the interests of the unit or mission. Furthermore, they are aware "as they approach actual fighting, [that] their autonomy dramatically decreases." Thus, when individuals join the military "they implicitly agree to subordinate their own interests and autonomy to the military when necessary for the unit or the mission." In response, the military promises "to protect them to the degree possible during combat."

In this context, the argument against allowing service members to grant or withhold informed consent becomes clear.

> If the military gave servicepersons the choice of accepting or refusing to take such compounds, those who chose not to take the compounds would violate the overriding obligation to the unit and the military, and the military would violate its obligation to them.

Those who refused could either leave the combat situation or remain without protection. The undesirable consequences would be to increase the danger to other service personnel, to reduce the likelihood of a successful mission, and potentially to place themselves at risk.

On the assumption that the benefits of taking the investigational compounds greatly exceed the risks, as evaluated as objectively as possible by civilian reviewers outside of DoD,

> permitting servicepersons to grant or withhold informed consent cannot be ethically justifiable *in principle* [emphasis in original] because this would give servicepersons' individual autonomy priority over their obligations to the unit and society, thus unnecessarily endangering other servicepersons and the success of the mission.

Two of the most prominent critics of the Interim Rule, Annas and Grodin, of Boston University, responded to Howe and Martin in the same issue of the *Hastings Center Report* (Annas and Grodin, 1991). They characterized the Interim Rule as a radical departure from long-standing DoD policy by requiring U.S. troops to take unapproved drugs and vaccines without consent—"informed or otherwise." That long-standing policy began in 1953, they argue, when DoD adopted the Nuremberg Code as official policy, including the essential requirement of informed consent for research subjects.[2] DoD policy had been consistent since 1953, then, and had included the adoption in 1986 of the "Proposed Model Federal Policy for the Protection of Human Subjects," which became the Common Rule.

Annas and Grodin rejected the argument that these policies were irrelevant because the INDs were being given for treatment not research. "Until now," they argued, the military position had been that service personnel "must accept standard medical treatment (or face court martial)." However, they have no obligation to accept interventions "not generally recognized as standard procedures." They quoted a decision of the Army Judge Advocate General that

> "only those [procedures] thoroughly tried and generally used by the medical professional that have definitely and finally passed the novel and experimental stages, and has been accepted as standard operations in surgery,"

can be performed without consent. The issue to Annas and Grodin was clear: "it is the experimental or investigational nature of the intervention, not the

---

[2]That policy, however, was classified as Top Secret until 1975, when then–U.S. Army Surgeon General Richard R. Taylor testified before a subcommittee of the U.S. Senate Judiciary Committee dealing with military experiments:

> The basic Department of Defense policy governing medical experiments was promulgated by the Secretary of Defense on 26 February 1953. This policy is based on the Nuremberg Code of 1947, which followed the war crimes trials. . . . [A]n individual participating as a subject is required to . . . give voluntary written informed consent without coercion. . . . These basic moral, ethical, and legal principles . . . are common to the regulations of the military departments.

intent [emphasis added] of the physician or researcher, that determines whether or not an intervention is research or therapy." Moreover, the absence of alternative treatments "does not convert an investigational intervention into a therapeutic one." Rather, consent is required for investigational drugs not only by the Nuremberg Code, but by the Declaration of Helsinki, HHS regulations, and FDA regulations.[3] Moreover, "*no exception* [emphasis in original] is made for the military or wartime in any of these codes and regulations."

Annas and Grodin attacked the DoD justifications for the Interim Rule. The argument that the investigational drugs used in the Gulf War were safe and effective and constituted the primary preventive treatment available was vitiated by DoD's request for an exception to use them without informed consent; if the interventions were treatments, no exemption and no consent would be required. Second, the second justification that consent was "not feasible" was basically an extension of Hippocratic paternalism from "the doctor knows best" to "the Army knows best" and represented a substantial assault on the rights of American servicemen and women. Third, service personnel do not subordinate themselves entirely to the military mission or to the welfare of their fellow soldiers. They have both a right and a duty to disobey an unlawful order. But was not the order to take investigational drugs the same as an order to wear protective clothing and equipment? "The answer is no," they responded.

> The helmet or flak jacket cannot injure the serviceperson, has no side effects, and can only protect. The unproven vaccine, on the other hand, can actually cause more problems than it solves and can cause more injury to individual troops than the biological agent it is designed to protect against.

They extended their argument even further: "Ground troops are not asked if they want to advance; they are ordered to advance even if many of them will likely perish. But the order to march does not justify the order to submit to experimental vaccines."

Finally, Annas and Grodin argued, in response to the DoD argument that the Nuremberg Code and the Declaration of Helsinki did not apply "to the wartime military," the Nuremberg Code was not articulated for the expedient purposes of "any country, army, or research endeavor." Rather, its principles

> were derived from [quoting the Code] "the principles of the law of nations as they result from the usages established among civilized peoples, from the laws of humanity, and from the dictates of public conscience." Those who fight to protect these basic human rights should be protected by them.

---

[3]Annas and Grodin were either unaware that FDA regulations allowed exceptions or chose to ignore this fact.

Also in the *Hastings Center Report*, Levine (1991) of Yale University School of Medicine, long-time student of institutional review boards and informed consent, thanked Howe and Martin for their "careful account of the ethical justifications" behind the interim final rule. He took up "the allegation" that DoD's planned use of investigational drugs was research. He cited the Belmont Report's definition of research as "an activity designed to test a hypothesis, permit conclusions to be drawn, and thereby to develop or contribute to generalizable knowledge" and that of DHHS regulations "as a systematic investigation designed to develop generalizable knowledge." The intended uses of INDs in the Gulf clearly did not constitute research but were intended to treat or prevent the "horrific" injuries that might be caused by chemical or biological warfare agents. These uses conformed to the definition of medical practice of the Belmont Report and also noted that the U.S. District Court had dismissed *Doe v. Sullivan*, in part, because of the "lack of conformity to the definition of research—within the meaning intended or specified in any relevant law." The frequent failure of many commentators to make the distinction between research and treatment stemmed, in Levine's view, from "incautious use of poorly defined terms and concepts" by many discussants. *Investigational*, in its denotative meaning, is applied to drugs not approved by FDA for commercial distribution; however, it connotes "images of research." Moreover, the term "investigational new drug" evolved within FDA from the *legal exemption* authorizing distribution across state boundaries for purposes of the conduct of research and only later came to refer to the drug or vaccine itself.

On the informed consent requirement for human use of all investigational drugs, even if used for therapy outside of a research protocol, Levine reasoned that military personnel "in certain situations do not have the same rights to self-determination as civilians; they may not refuse therapies designed to maintain their effectiveness." So when DoD determined that INDs were the best preventive or therapeutic treatment against CW/BW agents, "administering them without informed consent would have been in accord with customary military procedure." In response to critics of the Interim Rule who claimed that it was "feasible" to obtain consent in the Gulf, Levine concurred that it would be "doable" in the "very limited sense" of obtaining 500,000 signatures on consent forms, but that it would not be "reasonable" or "suitable."

In 1994, as Congress increased its postwar interest in the Gulf War, Arthur Caplan, prominent University of Pennsylvania bioethicist and later a member of the PAC on Gulf War Veterans' Illnesses, testified before a Senate committee (1994). The issue of whether the use of investigational drugs and vaccines in the Gulf for CW/BW defense constituted research or treatment was a settled issue in his view. It was research. Research, he argued, was defined by intent: "The standing definition of research in American law looks to intent to define research. If a goal of undertaking and intervention with a human being is to generate new knowledge then that activity counts as research."

Although the conduct of research on military personnel was "most difficult" when "threatened with the prospect of war or . . . actually engaged in an armed conflict," Caplan testified, the standards for such research were clear. They derived from the Nuremberg Code, which had been "set down as a direct response to experiments conducted under conditions of war," and which made

> *no exception* [emphasis added] for research conducted in the context of war. . . .

> The enormously important goal of protecting the nation's security is not held to be a value that is so overriding as to obliterate the individual subjects' rights. The Code states clearly and unambiguously that everyone involved in research is to be so informed and that they are to have the right to give or withhold their consent to that research.

The essential requirement of informed consent, Caplan argued, "is not modulated by the existence of a state of war."

Although some military efforts were clearly research, Caplan acknowledged that the military use in the Gulf War of PB and BT was arguably to protect troops from lethal chemical and biological agents and thus not research. For Caplan, these arguments were "not persuasive." Why? For one thing, he asserted, the use of "unapproved, unlicensed agents clearly" was understood by FDA and DoD to be research in that both agencies recognized the need to seek waivers from prevailing informed consent requirements. Moreover, it was understood by these regulatory and military officials that the practical reasons it was difficult to obtain consent "for the use of untested, unproven agents in large populations deployed in trying environments under battlefield conditions meant that the use of these agents had to be seen as experimental."

Although it could be argued that those seeking to use investigational agents to obtain prophylactic benefit for military personnel "did so by weighing carefully the cost, risk, and potential benefits," neither the conduct of such analysis, nor results of such analysis that favored the use of investigational agents, nor the intent to use such agents to "benefit, treat, or prevent harm" could "transform an experimental intervention into a therapy."

However, Caplan expressed reservation about this definition. Reliance on the regulatory definition of research as "intent to create generalizable knowledge" was fine as far as it went but it was not adequate to capture activities that are

> manifestly experimental but are not conducted with the intent of generating new knowledge. . . . This is obviously what took place in the Gulf with anti-bot toxoid [sic] and pyridostigmine bromide. These agents were used in large populations for purposes other than those for which they were originally designed in circumstances under which they had never before been tried.

Moreover, given uncertainty about what chemical or biological agents might have been deployed by Iraq, PB and BT "may have had no efficacy or might actually have had an adverse effect in the case of the utilization of certain nerve gas agents." Furthermore, efficacy was open to question in Caplan's view because the actual administration of these agents deviated from the normal three-shot regime (for BT). "It seems plain," he stated, that the most likely reason for the decision to grant the waiver was "that there was a chance the agents would do more good than harm but that the efficacy of these agents to prevent harm was seen as far from certain."

In the final paragraph of his testimony, Caplan offered this advice:

> Those engaged in decisions to use unproven, untested, unlicensed or otherwise experimental or research agents in the context of biological and chemical warfare or other battlefield circumstances must understand that conditions of war may lead to decisions which, while undertaken with the best of motives, may not serve to protect the welfare of military personnel or permit the completion of the assigned military mission. Americans when faced with a challenge often feel that it is better to try something rather than to do nothing. The history of human experimentation in this century shows that often, when faced with a crisis, doing nothing in the face of uncertainty can be the most prudent course of action to follow.

In summary, the critics make these arguments. First, they emphasize the unknowns of research. Annas and Grodin (1991), for example, state: "Research is research because we don't know the consequences, risks, and benefits of intervention." Caplan (1991) argues that the "manifestly experimental" nature of investigational drugs is clear because they "were used in large populations for purposes other than those for which they were originally designed in circumstances under which they had never before been tried."[4] Further, Caplan argues, the research nature of the use of PB and BT in the Gulf is "cemented by the obvious uncertainty that accompanied the utilization of these agents as to the efficacy that they would have in the field." Uncertainty about the consequences of nonuse in the face of enemy capabilities and intentions receives no attention.

Second, the critics attack the inadequacy of intent to differentiate between research and treatment. Here they rely on the Belmont Report as the authoritative statement that research is an activity whose purpose is to generate generalizable knowledge. Thus Caplan (1991) argues that, if intent were controlling "those who do research would merely have to change their intentions and they

---

[4]This view, taken to its logical conclusion, would classify early use of an FDA-approved drug as "experimental" because the small sample sizes in Phase I, II, and III clinical trials were inadequate to reveal rare side effects or long-term effectiveness in the intended population of normal users.

could succeed in making the most innovative and experimental medical interventions into therapies merely by a change of mind." In a similar vein, Annas
and Grodin (1991) write: "The point is clear. It is the experimental or investigational nature of the intervention, not the intent of the physician or
researcher, that determines whether or not an intervention is research or therapy." Both might have invoked Sabiston and Robertson at this juncture, neither
of whom found intent especially helpful. Also overlooked was the fact that few
advocates for the use of investigational drugs for CW/BW defense rely on intent
as the sole criterion differentiating between research and treatment, a matter
we discuss at greater length below.

Third, the critics argue that acceptance of the requirements of regulation constitutes de facto recognition that research is involved. Caplan testified: "The
use of unapproved, unlicensed agents was clearly understood by FDA and DoD
to be research inasmuch as both agencies recognized the need to seek waivers
from prevailing informed consent requirements." Such a categorical statement
denies the possibility that both parties might be proceeding on the basis that
ambiguity exists regarding the definition of research and that the relation
between *research* and *investigational* is an arguable policy issue, but that the
parties agree that deference should be given to established regulations even
while seeking to modify those regulations to accommodate challenges unanticipated when they were adopted. Martin (1996), responding to this point, said,
"Referring to these drugs and vaccines as "investigational" is in accordance
with Food and Drug Administration (FDA) regulations and is not a definitive
statement regarding the scientific information available about the INDs." In
addition, both Annas and Grodin, as well as Caplan, note that the Nuremberg
Code was conceived in the wake of war, both as a reaction to the despicable war
crimes of the Nazi doctors and as an effort to articulate "universal principles"
governing human experimentation. Then, since the code made *no exceptions*
for research in wartime, no exceptions should be tolerated for such situations as
the Gulf War. They reject as not pertinent the fact that the Nuremberg Code
was articulated with reference to a quite different empirical situation than that
existing in the Gulf in 1990 and 1991.

The purpose of the critics' line of argument is clear: If *investigational* means
research under any and all circumstances, informed consent is required at all
times. Consequently, a willingness to acknowledge that there may be distinc-
tions among various drugs FDA has classified as "investigational" is ruled out *a
priori*. In short, the experiment-therapy continuum does not represent a gray
zone for the critics, but investigational lies at all times on the research side of a
bright orange line.

If the weight of the *investigational* designation falls heavily on requiring
informed consent, how did DoD define both PB and BT as *treatment*, not

research, and justify waiving informed consent? The arguments, which were laid out in the Mendez letter of October 30, 1990, were as follows. First, DoD highlighted the Iraqi *threat* and the need to prepare in advance for the uncertainty of the enemy's capabilities and intentions. This was especially true for Saddam Hussein, who had previously used CW/BW agents in Iraq's war with Iran as well as against ethnic groups in Iraq itself. Second, there was the ethical commitment to protect U.S. military personnel from the threat that was at the heart of seeking approval to use "the best preventive or therapeutic treatment" available. Third, in scientific and clinical terms, the drugs under consideration, although classified by FDA as investigational, were not "exotic new drugs"; they were not novel. Rather, they had "well-established uses," both preventive and therapeutic. The DoD medical establishment had concluded that these drugs were the best available way to protect the troops. The safety of these drugs had been established by prior use, human data supported the effectiveness of BT and animal data provided a defensible scientific basis for the effectiveness of PB. Consequently, DoD was not proposing to engage in clinical investigation but to use these drugs as the only medical therapies available for the *treatment* (or pretreatment) of potentially lethal CW/BW agents. Hundreds of thousands of troops were at risk in the Gulf and the issue for DoD was how it should be fulfill its obligation to protect them, "How do we take care of people?"

In DoD's judgment, a gray zone existed in which products legally classified as investigational could be justifiably represented as having nonresearch, therapeutic uses. That gray zone was legally provided for in Section 505(i) of the FDCA. This section requires that investigators using drugs for investigational purposes

> inform any human beings to whom such drugs . . . are being administered, or their representatives, that such drugs are being used for investigational purposes and will obtain the consent of such human beings or their representatives, *except where they deem it not feasible or, in their professional judgment, contrary to the best interests of such human beings* [emphasis added].

This statutory provision for exceptions from the requirements of informed consent provides the basis for a "not feasible" determination and for DoD requesting waiver of informed consent of investigational drugs in the Gulf War.

FDA'S APPROACH TO THE DEFINITIONAL TASK

It is worth observing that FDA approaches the definitional task in a quite different manner. It actually makes no effort to define research per se. Instead, it refers to clinical investigations and emphasizes "adequate and well-controlled studies" as a requirement for approval of a drug. This requirement, in fact, presumes that one objective of such Phase III studies is therapeutic.

Most important, FDA places substantial weight on *methodology* as a defining feature of clinical investigations. Section 505(d) of the FDCA states that the secretary "shall refuse to approve" an [NDA] application if safety and effectiveness standards are not met. The criterion of "safe for use" is that a drug be supported by "adequate tests by all methods reasonably applicable"; the effectiveness criterion is that "substantial evidence that the drug will have the effect it purports or is represented to have" is met. *Substantial evidence* is further defined as

> evidence consisting of adequate and well-controlled studies, including clinical investigations, by experts qualified by scientific training and experience to evaluate the effectiveness of the drug involved, on the basis of which it could fairly and responsibly be concluded by such experts that the drug will have the effect it purports or is represented to have under the conditions of use prescribed, recommended, or suggested in the labeling or proposed labeling thereof.[5]

Thus, the FDCA, augmented by FDA regulations and guidelines, approaches the definition of clinical investigations not only with respect to *intent* but also with reference to statistical and clinical *methodology* and to the *qualifications of investigators* (which include both training and experience). This approach, constrained by the law, is far richer and more empirically grounded than that of the useful, but limited, Belmont Report.

---

[5]The importance of methodology, and of the quality of evidence as judged by experts qualified by training *and* experience to make scientific determinations, is sufficiently great that FDA's CDER has a 125-page *Guideline for the Format and Content of the Clinical and Statistical Sections of New Drug Applications*, published in 1988, which provides detailed instructions about reporting results of clinical investigations. In addition, this "guideline" requires that each NDA list "all investigators supplied with the drug substance or drug product by the applicant or known to have investigated the drug" and indicate the kinds of studies each investigator has conducted.

Chapter Four

THE INTERIM RULE AND ITS ALTERNATIVES

In this chapter, we deal analytically with the issues associated with the Interim Rule, focusing mainly on the "external" policy issues on which DoD requires the concurrence of FDA. However, we also consider those "internal" issues under the control of DoD, such as provision of information to military personnel about investigational drugs, whose implementation reflects on the merit of the general policy. In the first section, we consider the regulatory issues associated with the Interim Rule, as defined by the FDA's Request for Comments of July 31, 1997. Then, in the second section, we address three alternatives to the Interim Rule: revocation, "anticipatory consent," and other arrangements.

ISSUES ASSOCIATED WITH THE INTERIM RULE

Many, but not all, of the regulatory issues associated with the Interim Rule were raised in FDA's July 31, 1997, Request for Comments (62 FR 40966, July 31, 1997). Since the request constitutes the focus of rule making, and thus policy, the following discussion is organized in relation to the questions it asks. The request is organized by Questions A, B, and C: Question A asks eight numbered questions, of which the eighth has parts (a) through (g); Questions B and C ask about standards of approval. Most of these questions are discussed in this section. However, we consider the question about revocation of the rule (A-1) and the two questions about "anticipatory consent (A-4 and A-5) under "Alternatives to the Interim Rule" below. In addition, several questions are addressed in Chapter Five, "Broader Issues." Table 2 provides a guide to how the questions asked by FDA in its Request for Comments are considered in the text.

Question A-2 asks, "Are there circumstances under which the use of the Interim Rule would be justified? If so, what are those circumstances?" Several bioethicists, as noted above, answer this question with an absolutist position: The Nuremberg Code provides no basis for exceptions to informed consent on human subjects of research, and thus the Interim Rule is not justified. An abso-

Table 2

Guide to Discussion of Questions in FDA Request for Comments

Question	Subject of Question	Discussion in this Report
A	Interim Rule	
-1	Should the rule be revoked?	Alternatives to the Interim Rule
-2	Are there circumstances under which Interim Rule would be justified?	Regulatory Issues
-3	Is rationale for "not feasible" valid?	Broader Issues (Chapter Five)
-4	Anticipatory consent at recruitment	Alternatives to the Interim Rule
-5	Anticipatory consent in peacetime	Alternatives to the Interim Rule
-6	If Interim Rule is needed, what changes should be made?	Regulatory Issues
-7	Should Interim Rule be narrowed in scope?	General question answered in the details, including public comment
-8	"If the rule were to be reproposed: . . ."	
(a)	IRB independent of DoD	Regulatory Issues
(b)	Authority to make "not feasible" determination	Broader Issues (Chapter Five)
(c)	Information to military personnel: more specificity or more latitude?	Regulatory Issues
(d)	Information to military personnel: additional measures needed?	Regulatory Issues
(e)	Adequate record keeping	Regulatory Issues
(f)	Oversight and accountability	Broader Issues (Chapter Five)
(g)	Procedures to track noncompliance	Regulatory Issues
B	Standards of approval: testing toxic agents on human subjects	Regulatory Issues
C	Standards of approval: obtaining evidence of human efficacy	Regulatory Issues

lutist position, however, does not take into account the existence of foreign enemies, the possibilities such enemies might generate, the options appropriate for response, or the qualified nature of *investigational* that is invoked under the terms of the Interim Rule. As a factual matter, the possible use of CW/BW agents against U.S. military personnel in future conflicts cannot be ruled out. Neither can the possibility of thousands of American casualties be ruled out if medical treatment is not available among the several protective measures used against CW/BW agents. In such circumstances, the obligation of the U.S. military to its personnel is to protect individuals, ensure the safety of units, and maintain the military capability to conduct war. The use of investigational drugs for treatment, not research, to protect these personnel is justified, in our view, as is a policy authorizing waiver of informed consent for such use.

Two questions—A-3 and A-8(b)—ask about the feasibility of obtaining informed consent in certain military combat exigencies. Question A-3 asks the following:

> The Interim Rule is based on the premise that informed consent is not feasible in military combat exigencies because if a soldier were permitted to say "no," this could jeopardize the accomplishment of the combat mission. DoD has alleged that it is not an option to excuse a nonconsenting soldier from a military mission. Given the experience in the Gulf War, does this rationale still hold?

Question A-8(b) asks:

> Should the authority to make the "feasibility determination" (i.e., whether obtaining informed consent is "not feasible") under the Interim Rule be vested in persons or entities other than the Commissioner of FDA?

Both are addressed briefly below and at greater length in Chapter Five.

Question A-6 asks a general question: "If the Interim Rule is needed, are there changes that should be made to it based on experiences during and following the Gulf War? If so, what are these changes and why should they be made?" Our response deals with the issue of need and then with that of specific changes. First, the fact that DoD has concluded that the rule is needed should not be taken lightly: The military requested that the authority to waive informed consent be established in 1990; in 1991, after the Gulf War, it requested that rule making be completed and the Interim Rule made final; and it regards the Interim Rule as an important legal-regulatory policy today.

Looking backward, the needs of the military at the time of the Gulf War were: to proceed with adequate authorization, which meant not risking the creation ad hoc of an exclusively DoD-based authority but seeking the imprimatur of FDA; to have authorization tailored to perceived military requirements, i.e., with an exception from full compliance with FDA regulations; and to assure military personnel, including many civilian reservists, and the American public that it was taking its responsibilities to protect such personnel very seriously. Therefore, any negative answer to the question about need ought to argue, at the very least, that DoD is wrong *militarily.*

Second, the implications of a negative answer to this question are also discussed below under "Revocation." Revocation would not be a return to the pre–Interim Rule status, but would, instead, constitute a *denial* of the authority to waive informed consent for CW/BW defensive use of investigational drugs. A policy that progressed from silence to affirmation to negation (a reversal of affirmation) could create the possibility of a war-related controversy at some future time. In our view, this would be unfortunate if it forced a choice between protecting U.S. troops and complying with FDA regulations.

Regarding specific changes that might be made in the rule, many are discussed below. Question A-8, for example, asks the policy question, "If the rule were to be reproposed," then breaks this down into a number of specific questions; the greater part of this section is devoted to discussing these specific questions. Other questions, such as Question A-7, which asks, "Can or should the Interim Rule be narrowed in scope? If so, how?," are left for the rule-making process and specific recommended changes. Finally, the general issue of oversight and accountability asked by Question A-8(f), "Should the rule contain additional procedures to enhance understanding, oversight, and accountability? If so, what are these procedures?," is dealt with in Chapter Five.

Question A-8(a): IRB Independent of DoD.

Question A-8(a) asks about the IRB that is required under the Interim Rule to review and approve the use of an investigational drug without informed consent:

> Should there be a requirement that DoD's proposed use of the investigational product(s) be approved by an IRB that is independent of DoD? If so, why should DoD be held to a requirement not imposed on other institutions, and what should be the requirement for that independent IRB? Can this be accomplished without compromising military or national security? (Request for Comments.)

DoD, like all federal agencies supporting or conducting research, is required to adhere to the Common Rule regarding the protection of human subjects [45 CFR 46], which requires that "one or more" IRBs review and approve (or disapprove) research protocols involving human subjects. An IRB is required to consist of "at least five members, with varying backgrounds to promote complete and adequate review of research activities commonly conducted by the institution." Members are to reflect professional experience and expertise, diversity, and sensitivity to community attitudes; are not to be all of one gender or selected on the basis of gender; and are not to be of a single profession. The board must include at least one member whose primary concerns are scientific and one whose primary concerns are nonscientific and at least one member who is not affiliated with the institution and is not an immediate family member of an affiliated individual. No member may participate in a review in which he or she has a conflicting interest. The IRB may invite, at its discretion, nonvoting individuals with special competence to assist with reviews for which it lacks expertise.

Edgar and Rothman (1995), in a general review and critique of the IRB system unrelated to DoD, the Interim Rule, and ODS, ask, regarding the proliferation of such committees, "Is it truly the case that a 'one size fits all' approach works well?" They elaborate in the following way:

> Are the same general procedures for appointing members and defining their obligations appropriate for reviewing research conducted not only at the

Central Intelligence Agency (CIA), the Bureau of Prisons, and the National Institutes of Health (NIH), but also at for-profit hospitals, local community hospitals, and university-affiliated tertiary-care centers? Does it make sense to give the leadership of an institution, which by its very nature cannot survive without the funds and fame brought in by clinical research, the responsibility for appointing the membership of a monitoring committee?

The intent of the Edgar and Rothman critique is to suggest that the answer to the above questions is no and to make some modest recommendations for change. They indicate that FDA oversight of IRB decisions provides "a degree of national oversight for clinical research." But they basically conclude that "the power to approve or disapprove research on ethical grounds is granted to a local institutional committee," that "no federal controls or regulations exist on how the institution decides who gets appointed to the committee, how long those persons stay, or on what grounds a member may be dismissed or not reappointed," that there is "no strong framework to ensure that subjects' interests take precedence over institutional ones," and that "there are very few provisions in the regulations that protect against bodies that might be sloppy, venal, or subservient to the institution." (Edgar and Rothman, 1995, pp. 492, 493.)

After reviewing the history of medical experimentation that abused human subjects, and the resultant conclusion that review by a body other than the investigator was necessary to ensure ethical treatment of such subjects, Edgar and Rothman review the assumptions underlying the dependence on *local* IRBs. They find all of them to be less compelling today, criticize continued reliance on "one size fits all," and make the following recommendations. First, they argue that "public visibility" and time for "political choice" are required to protect the public "from the ends [i.e., objectives] of research" and the development of new medical technologies and that a *national* monitoring system of a "super" committee or committees ought to be considered. Second, they argue that the newly entrepreneurial character of academic medical research raises conflict-of-interest questions that are "the appropriate object for formal legal rules." Third, they recommend that reform should "strengthen the 'outside' elements of IRBs, while leaving the review based in the institution itself." Finally, they recommend "far more effective oversight mechanisms" than currently exist.

This critique by Edgar and Rothman of reliance on local IRBs is cited for two reasons. First, it makes clear that there are enough questions of public policy importance to justify a thorough and overarching review of the *entire* system. Indeed, this is perhaps the main reason the National Bioethics Advisory Committee was created. Second, the Edgar and Rothman review is directed to the *research* enterprise, not to situations in which treatment is the primary issue. Thus, the applicability of their critique to the DoD situation in ODS is a matter deserving independent consideration.

In the case of the Gulf War, the review by an IRB of the waivers requested under the Interim Rule was described by Dr. Edward Martin, then Principal Deputy ASD(HA), in testimony to the Presidential Advisory Committee on Gulf War Veterans' Illnesses:

> The Department of Defense (DoD) IRB review for ODS was accomplished through The Army Surgeon General's Human Subjects Research Review Board (HSRRB). The HSRRB was established in 1975, replacing the review functions of three other committees which existed at that time: the Army Investigational Drug Review Board, the Contract Review Board, and the Clinical Investigations Committee. The HSRRB is administered by the Human Use Review and Regulatory Affairs Division (HURRAD) of the U.S. Army Medical Research and Materiel Command. The HURRAD was established in 1974 as the Human Use Review Office during the same time frame that the Office for Protection from Research Risks (OPRR) was established at the National Institutes of Health (NIH). The HURRAD performs similar functions for the Office of The Army Surgeon General (OTSG) as does the OPRR for NIH. The HSRRB acts for OTSG as an IRB, ethics advisory board and human research policy board. The HSRRB recommends protocols for approval by OTSG and may also recommend revisions to, or disapproval of, protocols. The HSRRB provides both a second level IRB review and acts as the sole IRB for selected protocols, especially those from institutions which do not have their own IRB, or for contingency or mobilization type protocols. The Army serves as the DoD executive Agent for Biological and Chemical Defense Programs.

> At the time of ODS, the HURRAD and the HSRRB were well experienced in the regulatory processes and the ethics of the human subject experience with INDs.[1] The Acting Chairman of the HSRRB at that time was a physician with approximately ten years experience as Acting Chairman. The HSRRB acted as the sole IRB in this case to centralize the process for several different INDs coming from different sources. In the situation with ODS, the HSRRB acted for the Army, the Army being the DoD Executive Agent for the Biological and Chemical Defense Programs.

> The HSRRB and later the FDA deliberated these ethical issues on each individual IND on a case-by-case basis. The medical risks versus the benefits of using the specific INDs were weighed against the risks of not using the INDs. The primary decision put before the HSRRB was whether or not the autonomy of an individual Service member to make his/her own decision outweighed the need to protect that Service member and/or fellow Service members in potentially life-threatening situations. Based on the long history of human use of the approved drug, Pyridostigmine Bromide (MestinonR), and also that of the IND Botulinum Toxoid vaccine, and the human safety and animal efficacy, these INDs were determined to be the best medical protective measures available

---

[1]This quotation does not distinguish between an IND, which is the *application* to test an investigational drug, and the *drug* itself. It is clear from the context that reference is to the latter.

against the threat of potential exposure to certain nerve agents and botulinum toxins. The HSRRB recommend the approval of the use of these two products for medical pretreatment and prophylaxis without the requirement of informed consent. The FDA required the epidemiological follow-up for collecting adverse event data, where possible. These recommendations represented the best medical treatment decisions at the time for the protection of our Service men and women. (Martin, 1996.)

We return then to the FDA question of why it might be argued that DoD should have an "independent" IRB. We may infer an answer, namely, that those advocating an "independent" IRB hold that an IRB organized under the auspices of the DoD cannot be trusted to implement the laws and regulations for the protection of human subjects faithfully. A more likely argument for an IRB independent of DoD rests on the belief that an *institutional conflict of interest* exists for such an IRB and that this conflict either renders it incapable of impartial judgment or unable to allay concern about impartiality. Such a conflict, actual or perceived, might lead members of a DoD IRB, when INDs are proposed for use to protect troops from lethal CW/BW agents, to give greater weight to a request to waive informed consent for treatment purposes than to protecting military personnel in the context of *human research subjects.* On the other hand, a DoD IRB is likely to spend most of its time reviewing research protocols and consent forms for projects that are identical to civilian research projects and only infrequently to be asked to review a waiver of informed consent request under the Interim Rule.

Financial conflict of interest is the threat to impartiality of judgment that Edgar and Rothman suggest is the institutional conflict likely to confront academic IRBs in the contemporary world of biomedicine. The latter is addressed only by the requirement that there be one IRB member who has no ties to the institution in question, a very weak protection. More complicated is the conflict of interest stemming from *intellectual bias.* This matter was addressed briefly in an Institute of Medicine study (1992) of FDA advisory committees several years ago, in which such conflict was described as "the subtly and perhaps even overtly biasing effects on objectivity of a scientist's prior research and public positions, particularly positions taken in formal administrative or judicial proceedings." This area, however, is essentially uncharted territory, and the issues that might arise here are hardly any different in the military than in a civilian context.

Substantively, the IRB question in a Gulf War–type situation is precisely that posed by Martin in his PAC testimony:

> The medical risks versus the benefits of using the specific INDs were *weighed against the risks of not using the INDs* [emphasis added]. The primary decision put before the HSRRB was whether or not the autonomy of an individual Ser-

vice member to make his/her own decision outweighed the need to protect that Service member and/or fellow Service members in potentially life-threatening situations. (Martin, 1996)

The argument for an IRB independent from DoD may turn on whether one believes that taking the risk of enemy use and the consequences of enemy use of lethal chemical and biological weapons into account is appropriate. Should the scope of IRB deliberations be limited to the risks and benefits of using the investigational drug, or should it also include the risks of nonuse? It could be argued that a DoD IRB is more likely to include members with expertise related to the broader issue of the risk nonuse than an independent IRB focused more narrowly on a risk-benefit analysis of the drug.

Assume for this discussion that a judgment is reached favoring an independent IRB on the grounds that a DoD IRB is incapable of impartial judgment when confronted with a request for waiver of informed consent under the Interim Rule. There are then a number of complicated questions to be addressed, including the appointing authority (the FDA Commissioner, the Secretary of Health and Human Services, the President?), the criteria for selection of members (no veterans, some veterans, former enlisted men, former officers, all civilians with no prior military service, and what other kinds of expertise?), and the circumstances that would trigger the convening of this extraordinary IRB (after a congressional declaration of war, a presidential declaration of emergency?). In the last analysis, an independent IRB does not resolve the need to appoint human beings to exercise their best judgment about vexing issues in time of national emergency.

In the Gulf War situation, there is no evidence that the DoD IRB was not in compliance with all pertinent laws and regulations of the FDA and the DHHS regarding protection of human subjects. Even if such evidence existed, are there no remedies short of creating an independent IRB? Perhaps, following Edgar and Rothman, oversight might be strengthened; the members might be reminded of their obligations to uphold the law; and, if necessary, sanctions might be brought against them or against the IRB. Or perhaps several outside members, drawn from a pool of experts identified by DHHS and FDA, could be selected to ensure that the IRB does not subordinate its judgment to actual or perceived preferences of military authority. In any event, such remedies should be explored, as a policy based solely on distrust provides little basis for arguing for an IRB that is independent of DoD.

However, if distrust should prevail and provide a policy basis for establishing an independent IRB, could a policy be adopted that would leave *any institution,* whether a department or agency of the federal government or a research university, immune from challenge that it was unable to exercise impartial judgment because of institutional conflict of interest. Here we return to the general critique Edgar and Rothman developed. A recent congressional hearing (U.S. House, 1997) took several DHHS agencies—the NIH, CDC, and FDA—to task for research that did not adequately protect human subjects. Interestingly enough, the Director of OPRR was not present at that hearing, suggesting an institutional interest in his absence. Similarly, the scientific literature and popular press report from time to time on experimentation at universities that suggests lax IRB review or that the IRB might be subject to undue influence by prominent academic investigators. If a special rule requiring an independent IRB is crafted for DoD, why not apply the same logic to other federal agencies or to universities that stray from sanctioned behavior? In this context, one might also ask why the OPRR, a regulatory entity, is housed in the Office of the Director of the NIH, an agency whose primary mission is to support and conduct scientific research.

In short, any number of institutional conflict-of-interest questions might be raised, only some of which would apply to DoD. All human institutions are second best, including IRBs. Treating DoD separately from other agencies, absent compelling evidence of noncompliance with law and regulations, appears to be driven, in part, by an ill-defined search for a "best" arrangement without regard for the implications for all other "second-best" arrangements.

Question A-8(b): Determination That Informed Consent Is "Not Feasible"

The second question asked with reference to the potential reproposal of the Interim Rule pertains to who should make the determination that obtaining informed consent is not feasible in certain military exigencies. The question reads:

> Should the authority to make the "feasibility determination" i.e., whether obtaining informed consent is "not feasible") under the interim rule be vested in persons or entities other than the Commissioner of FDA? [Request for Comments]

The Interim Rule [21 CFR 50.23(d)] is one of *three exceptions* to the general requirements for informed consent. The first exception to the requirement of informed consent is provided by 21 CFR 50.23(a), which may be used when the investigator and a physician "not otherwise participating in the clinical investigation" certify in writing *all* of the following: that the human subject confronts a "life-threatening situation" necessitating the use of the investigational product in question; that informed consent cannot be obtained due to "an inability to communicate with, or obtain legally effective consent from, the subject"; that time is "not sufficient" to obtain consent from the subject's legal representative;

and that there is "no alternative method of approved or generally recognized therapy" providing an equal or greater probability of saving the subject's life. This exception is qualified by 21 CFR 50.23(b), which authorizes use of an investigational intervention if its immediate use, in the investigator's opinion, is "required to save the life of the subject, and time is not sufficient to obtain [in advance] the independent determination" required in (a) above. In such cases, the investigator's determinations shall be "reviewed and evaluated in writing by a physician who is not participating in the clinical investigation" within five working days.

The Interim Rule provides the second exception in a way that is more specific, formal, and less subject to abuse. The language of the Interim Rule states that the commissioner may determine that obtaining informed consent is not feasible

> when the Assistant Secretary of Defense (Health Affairs) requests such a determination in connection with the use of an investigational drug (including an antibiotic or biological product) in a specific protocol under an investigational new drug application (IND) sponsored by the Department of Defense (DoD).

This request must "be limited to a specific military operation involving combat or the immediate threat of combat"; it must also include written justification by the physicians responsible for care of the military personnel that

> to facilitate the accomplishment of the military mission, preservation of the health of the individual and the safety of other personnel require that a particular treatment be provided to a specified group of military personnel, *without regard to what might be any individual's personal preference* [emphasis added] for no treatment or for some alternative treatment

and that a "duly constituted" IRB has reviewed the use of the investigational drug without informed consent. In addition, the rule states that the commissioner "may find that informed consent is not feasible only when withholding treatment would be contrary to the best interests of military personnel and there is no available satisfactory alternative therapy."

A third exception [21 CFR 50.24], adopted in 1996, authorizes the waiver of informed consent for emergency use. The extensive deliberations surrounding this exceptions are set out in great detail in the NPRM (60 FR 49086, September 21, 1995) and in the final rule (61 FR 51498, October 2, 1996). Parenthetically, the deliberative process followed in this case may provide a model for the DoD-FDA consultation discussed below.

The first and third exceptions derive from life-threatening *individual* emergencies. In these cases, the commissioner is acting with respect to clinical situations that arise, however infrequently, in the familiar context of civilian medical care. The meaning of "not feasible" in this context is "not technically possible." The exception provided by the Interim Rule, however, flows from a *national security* emergency, not an individual emergency. In the situation addressed by the Interim Rule, "not feasible" goes beyond "not technically possible" to mean that it is not feasible to obtain informed consent and maintain military discipline.

Largely unspoken in official documents and discussions, but hardly unimportant, "not feasible" also has an *intelligence* dimension within the national security context. It was argued, for example, that General Schwarzkopf did not disclose in advance to General Belihar, his Command Surgeon, the identity of the military units that were to receive the anthrax and botulinum toxoid vaccines. This information was withheld to protect against the possibility that such "order of battle" information might be transmitted to the Iraqis and thus might identify to the enemy those units designated for the advance attack group. How would such information be obtained and conveyed? It takes little imagination to develop a scenario in which Iraqi informers were operating in and around coalition forces in Saudi Arabia for the express purpose of obtaining intelligence. So "not feasible" in the Gulf War context not only goes beyond "not technically possible" to embrace the issue of military discipline but, further, implies strategic considerations of an intelligence nature.

The question, then, of whether the FDA Commissioner should make the "not feasible" decision needs to be disaggregated into three distinct parts: DoD compliance with the requirements of the FDCA; FDA determination of *medical* aspects of "not feasible"; and DoD determination of *military* aspects of "not feasible." More specifically,

- The compliance issue stems from the facts that FDCA governs the use of investigational drugs, that DoD acknowledges FDA's authority in this regard, and that DoD has found it necessary to obtain FDA's determination that its actions under the Interim Rule were not in violation of the FDCA.

- The medical feasibility issues that the FDA Commissioner is clearly qualified to address include the safety and effectiveness of a drug, the "context" in which it will be administered, the nature of the disease or condition for which it will be used, and the information to be provided to a drug's recipients about "the potential benefits and risks of taking or not taking the drug."

- The military feasibility issues that DoD is most qualified to address include the risk of adverse health effects if lethal CW/BW agents are used; the military intelligence assessment of the probability that such agents will be used; the appropriate response, both military and ethical, to uncertainty about use of such agents; considerations about who in the chain of command makes what decisions regarding use of investigational drugs for CW/BW defensive purposes; and the battlefield impact of requiring consent.

The Interim Rule as currently written is explicit with respect to compliance with FDCA and the appropriateness of the FDA Commissioner making the determination about the medical elements of "not feasible." But it is much less explicit regarding how the military aspects of "not feasible" are determined. Clarification of the respective roles and responsibilities of DoD and the FDC Commissioner is warranted with respect to this matter, with one possible modification to the current rule being a procedure that involves joint determination that informed consent is not feasible in medical and military terms.

Question A-8(c) and A-8(d): Information to Military Personnel

Two questions are asked in the Request for Comments about the provision of information to military personnel, and by extension, to civilian DoD and contractor personnel in theaters of operations. The rule itself simply states that the Commissioner, in reaching a determination that informed consent is not feasible, shall "take into account [inter alia] . . . the nature of the information to be provided to the recipients of the drug concerning the potential benefits and risks of taking or not taking the drug." The first of the two questions [A-8(c)], then, asks

> Should the rule be more specific in describing the information that must be supplied to military personnel, or should FDA have wide latitude to make such determinations on a case-by-case basis? [Request for Comments]

The second question [A-8(d)] appears to lack a referent for "additional measures" but presumably refers to A-8(c) regarding the specificity of the rule versus the discretionary latitude to FDA. It asks

> Should additional measures be taken to insure that information required by FDA is effectively conveyed to the affected military personnel? If so, in what way? [Request for Comments]

There is no question that the failure to provide adequate information to military personnel with respect to PB and the BT and AX vaccines was a serious failure of DoD in the Gulf War in complying with the Interim Rule. Although pressures of time can explain much of the problem in the Gulf, the problem is one that clearly must be remedied with respect to the future.

With respect to the above questions, three things can be said. First, a final rule could usefully indicate a requirement that any request for a waiver under the rule be accompanied by DoD submission of the information that it proposes to provide to military and appropriate civilian personnel. It could also include a feature for DoD reporting back to FDA on the experience. Such a declarative statement should be general and brief, leaving the details to be addressed in a specific situation.

Second, in general, for certain investigational products, such as those used in the Gulf, the information requirements can conceivably be addressed separately from a specific IND. In Chapter Five, under "DoD-FDA Interactions," the argument is developed that a range of general issues should be addressed in ways that are not subordinate to particular applications. The FDA regulatory process, as suggested earlier, has developed over more than three decades with respect to the commercial pharmaceutical industry. If DoD use, or prospective use, of investigational drugs, differs from commercial drug development in important ways, as we believe it does, then it is worth considering a more systematic process for dealing with general issues as opposed to specific applications.

Third, with respect to "additional measures," the equivalent of a checklist of such measures might be indicated in the rule, with the details left for specification in direct interaction between FDA and DoD in the review of specific applications. This would be prescriptive as to additional measures to be considered but discretionary as to content.

Pendergast, in her testimony of July 29, 1997, before the Presidential Advisory Committee, indicated that FDA was considering a conference focused on special topics as part of its rule-making process. Later, we argue that such a conference should be held; here we simply argue that the question of information to military and appropriate civilian personnel should be one item on the agenda of such a conference.

Question A-8(e): Adequate Record Keeping

The failure to provide adequate record keeping with respect to PB and the BT and AX vaccines was also a very serious problem for DoD in the Gulf War. Although pressures of time and the chaos of war can explain much of the problem in the Gulf War, the matter is clearly one that must be remedied for the future. The Request for Comments asks:

> Should the rule address what constitutes adequate recordkeeping and adequate long-term follow-up of individuals who receive investigational products? If so, in what way? [Request for Comments]

Again, a final rule could usefully indicate a requirement that any waiver request under the rule be accompanied by DoD record keeping plan, or by compelling justification that a theater of operations does not permit good record keeping.

Such a requirement should be general and brief, with details addressed in a specific situation.

Furthermore, record keeping is a topic that could be considered in the conference that FDA has indicated it might hold as part of the current rule making. It is also a matter for continuing discussion between DoD and FDA, independent of a specific application for a waiver.

Question A-8(g): Procedures to Track Noncompliance

The Request for Comments asks "Should the rule contain additional procedures to track noncompliance?" The language might better be stated as "whether the rule should contain additional procedures to ensure compliance." Apart from semantic considerations, the issue here, once again, is how detailed the rule should be beyond a general declaration of a requirement and how much should be left to administrative discretion, on the grounds that the future cannot be anticipated, with respect to a waiver request by DoD and the response by FDA.

Standards of Approval

At the substantive heart of the Request for Comments, and of any submission of an IND or NDA by DoD and of the criteria for review of any application by FDA, are the standards of approval for an application. The request asks the following two questions:

> *Question B.* "When is it ethical to expose volunteers to toxic chemical and biological agents to test the effectiveness of products that may be used to provide potential protection against those agents?" [Request for Comments]

> *Question C.* "If products that may be used to provide potential protection against toxic chemical and biological agents cannot be ethically tested in humans, what evidence would be needed to demonstrate their safety and effectiveness?" [Request for Comments]

The scientific and clinical issues surrounding Questions B and C are beyond the scope of this paper. Nevertheless, a few comments are in order. The response to Question B from DoD, and from many other disinterested parties, has been that it is never ethical to expose volunteers to lethal chemical or biological agents in a clinical trial designed to test the effectiveness of prophylactic measures. The informed consent requirement makes the likelihood that individuals will volunteer to participate very low, and consent would be open to challenge in any event. More pertinent, the risk to individuals from exposure to such agents is too great to be countenanced. Even if dosage or exposure were reduced to tolerable levels, the results would be unlikely to be informative.

However, FDA clearly regards Question B as a serious scientific-clinical and ethical question and one that pertains not only to the situation raised by the threat of CW/BW agents in active military conflict but also to products that might be used to protect against hazardous industrial chemical and biological materials in occupational settings. Notwithstanding the FDA's position, DoD has answered Question B with a strong negative for the above reasons, leaving aside the storm of political criticism that would greet any other response.

DoD and FDA are addressing the scientific and clinical issues regarding Question C in relation to a BLA in the case of the BT vaccine and in relation to an NDA for PB. The general issue, however, deserves consideration should FDA decide to hold a conference as part of the current rule-making process.

ALTERNATIVES TO THE INTERIM RULE

The question of alternatives to the Interim Rule was raised initially in the Final Report of the PAC, but is addressed again in the FDA's July 31, 1997,[2] Request for Comments, which asked the following three questions, each of which is addressed below.

- "Should the agency *revoke* [emphasis added] the interim rule? If so, why?"

- "Instead of waiving the requirement for informed consent, is it feasible to obtain *anticipatory consent* [emphasis added] from military personnel during peace time for the future use of investigational products during a military conflict? If it is feasible, would such consent be valid as 'informed consent'? What would be the needed consent algorithm to make it valid and feasible."

- "Instead of waiving the requirement for informed consent, is it feasible to obtain *anticipatory consent* [emphasis added] from military recruits (prior to their recruitment into the military) for the future use of investigational products during a military conflict? If it is feasible, would such consent be valid? What would be the needed consent algorithm to make it valid and feasible."

Revocation

The FDA Request for Comments asks about revoking the Interim Rule in its entirety. The difficulties of this prospective approach can be understood more clearly if placed in the following historical context. First, in the period before ODS, no explicit authority existed that would allow the FDA Commissioner to

---

[2]In the period since this report was written, legislative developments have made this discussion moot. See the Postscript for a summary of those developments.

waive, or even to review a request for a waiver of, the informed consent requirement for the use of investigational drugs in certain military combat exigencies. Then, with the Interim Rule of December 21, 1990, explicit authority to do just that was established. Now, should the Interim Rule be revoked, such action would constitute explicit denial of previously established need.

What would the implications of revocation be? That depends on how FDA chose to take such a step. If revocation was accompanied by a statement that FDA requirements, which were not developed for military contingencies, did not apply in circumstances like those of the Gulf War, DoD might have a freer hand to respond within the context of the military contingencies it confronted. If, on the other hand, FDA stated or implied that there would be no exemptions from FDA requirements, even for CW/BW agents in a Gulf War situation, that would be potentially dangerous.

If in such a situation, PB and BT vaccine were, as in 1990, the best available preventive and therapeutic drugs available for defensive purposes, even though investigational, the question would confront the President in his role as Commander in Chief. This scenario, in our judgment, is one that we believe should be avoided. We return to this issue at greater length below.

Anticipatory Consent

The fundamental purpose that the military confronts in all of this is to address the question of how to protect military forces. This purpose should be kept clearly in mind in the discussion below.

The FDA Request for Comments asks about two forms of *anticipatory consent*, an undefined form of consent that currently does not exist in statute or regulation. These two forms are, first, consent by military personnel during peacetime and, second, consent before recruitment into the military. We consider anticipatory consent with reference to three potential situations, which embrace the FDA's two situations: consent at recruitment, consent during basic training, and consent before deployment to a theater of operations where the prospect of active conflict or exposure to CW/BW toxins is high.

The analysis of anticipatory consent is addressed with respect to the following issues: a plausible scenario for the situation; implications of the timing of the request; the scope or range of investigational products for which consent is sought; the duration that consent is presumed to be valid; and the effect of refusal of consent.

In general, the *timing* of the request for consent is the characteristic that differentiates informed consent as it is currently understood from the undefined anticipatory consent. The principal unknown is what is the effect of divorcing consent from the actual moment of decisionmaking. One can hypothesize the following effects on an individual's decision under such circumstances: The individual subject dismisses the significance of the decision to consent because it bears no direct relationship to actual conflict; fear is induced in the individual and overrides reason regarding risks and benefits, simply because the potential intervention is described as investigational; subtle (or not so subtle) coercion occurs in the way consent is sought; or information is provided to military personnel in an unbalanced way, in a setting that does not encourage individuals to ask questions of others, or in a way that does not stimulate discussion among troops.

Closely related to timing is the question of the *content* of the information that is provided to service personnel. How are the risks and benefits of an investigational drug to be presented in relation to the risk of an enemy's potential use of CW/BW agents? Should the risk-benefit calculation restrict itself to a civilian context of risk of investigational drug versus no treatment, and rule out consideration of enemy threat, or should it also include consideration of such a threat?

If an enemy threat is to be considered, are all potential enemies to be included, or only some, the most probable? Or is consent to a hypothetical conflict sufficient? If enemy capabilities and intentions are assessed at the time consent is given, what might the content of such information include, say, in April 1990 with respect to Saddam Hussein and Iraq?

The issue of *scope* or range of investigational products to which military personnel might be asked to give consent for use is also not straightforward if the consent decision is divorced from the actual situation. Should military personnel be asked about *all* investigational products that are in the DoD pipeline at the time of asking—drugs, vaccines, and medical devices? or only those that are most likely to be used? On what basis might a distinction be made between all and some? Should consent be obtained for all, for some, or only for the "most probable," however defined? Do self-administered products pose issues that differ from medic-administered products?

The question of the *duration* for which consent is valid is also complicated. The Interim Rule restricts waivers granted under it to a maximum of 12 months or cessation of conflict, whichever comes first. If a decision to consent is given at any time other than close to deployment, for how long is it valid? for the entire tour of duty? for three years? for one year? A consideration that is related to duration and timing also bears on scope: What are the implications of obtaining consent about a set of investigational products at a time when no alternative therapies exist, if things change and—at deployment—a better therapy has emerged, but is itself still investigational?

Finally, there is the issue of the effect of *refusal to consent*. Under normal civilian circumstances, there is no penalty to an individual who refuses to provide consent. In a military situation, however, might an individual be allowed to "join the military" and then, by refusing to consent to the use of investigational drugs, be exempted from service in the war-fighting part of the military?

We next consider each of the three possibilities for obtaining consent—at recruitment, in basic training, and at time of deployment to an active or potentially active theater of operations—in relation to the above questions.

Anticipatory Consent at Time of Recruitment. One plausible scenario might occur in the recruiting office of a military service. Recruiters are available at specified hours to interview individuals who come in to discuss joining the military. Another scenario might involve the recruiter visiting a high school or college campus to interview prospective candidates. Neither recruiters nor potential recruits have any illusions about the encounter: Both expect that information will be provided to the potential recruit; but both also understand that the recruiter's purpose is clearly to obtain enlistments.

This "before enlistment" situation appears quite problematic for obtaining informed consent for the use of investigational drugs. The situation is confounded by the fact that the U.S. military is today an all-volunteer military, conscription having been confined to the history books for the present time. The decision by an individual to enlist, coupled with military efforts to recruit, is a contractual decision when compared to conscription. The reasons for voluntarily joining the military range from a desire "to grow up," to obtain discipline, to obtain education, to learn an occupational specialty for a postmilitary career, or to seek a military career. For the individual, a decision to join the military involves *a priori* acceptance of the possibility that he or she might be placed in harm's way.

One can only speculate about the likely effects of seeking consent under such circumstances. Is the desire to join the military likely to override concerns about the hypothetical possibility that one might be asked to take investigational drugs? Or are individuals more likely to rethink and turn away from a decision to join? Problems arise in either direction.

Moreover, military recruiters may not be the most appropriate persons in whom DoD should vest the responsibility to explain the risks and benefits of investigational drugs. They probably lack the educational training that would equip them to provide good information and explanations. Their defined role is to recruit. Thus, they are likely to minimize risk in favor of obtaining another recruit. It is also not feasible, to take an alternative possibility, for medics to sit at recruitment offices.

Finally, consent at this stage would be to some hypothetical conflict situation and with respect to the then-current state of research knowledge about certain investigational products. It is difficult to regard this as informed, and it is clearly quite different from informed consent in the civilian context.

The *scope* of the consent requested is also problematic, as the questions and discussion above suggest. Absent a consent decision that is related in real time to the actual possibility of conflict, there is no apparent way to obtain consent for some investigational products but not for all. What is quite likely, however, is that only some products will be relevant in an actual conflict situation but that these will be known only in relation to that situation. Moreover, the differences between self-administered and medic-administered drugs may enter here.

The *duration* of a valid consent is also a complicated issue. It is difficult to believe that consent obtained at recruitment would withstand challenge, including possible legal challenges, at the time active or potentially active conflict was under consideration.

Finally, the effect of *refusal to consent*, if it carried no penalty, would provide an incentive for those who wished to benefit from military service but to do so without accepting the danger inherent in such service. This seems a pernicious set of incentives for organizing the military, given the dubious benefits of the approach. If refusal to consent meant, however, that an individual could not join unless they signed a consent form, they might respond, "OK, I'll sign anything to get in." In which case, the issue of coercion arises.

Anticipatory Consent During Basic Training. Many of the concerns expressed above about obtaining consent pertain to the basic training situation. However, basic training does have the advantage of being a good period during which information about the subject of chemical and biological warfare threats and countermeasures, including medical countermeasures, can be usefully introduced to military personnel in education and training sessions. If such information is part of training, hypotheticals are quite appropriate, and the scope can be comprehensive with respect to both threats and countermeasures. The issues of duration and the effects of refusal need not arise if consent is not sought. The crowded basic training schedule may make this option infeasible.

Anticipatory Consent Before Deployment. Of the three anticipatory approaches, this is the most attractive. The timing of the request for consent would be related to the actual situation of threat and current status of investigational products. (This begs the question, however, of how to define "before deployment," a nontrivial issue.) The scope would be limited to products actively being considered for use. The duration would similarly be limited to the specific conflict situation or to a 12-month period.

However, several problems exist with this approach. First, the question regarding the use of investigational drugs for CW/BW defense is the precise timing of administration. PB is self-administered and was handed out at the unit level to be taken in advance of an expected attack on orders of the unit commander. In the predeployment situation, when is consent to be obtained? on introduction to the theater? for each packet? or when a confirmed incoming Scud missile believed to be carrying nerve agent is confirmed? In the last case, a field commander is likely to respond on short notice with the command to "Take your medicine," especially if a drug such as PB with reversible effects is involved. Vaccines differ, since these are typically administered by field medics and require a period of time for immunity to develop. The full anthrax dose requires six shots over 18 months, three in the first six weeks and three more at six-month intervals, although DoD is seeking to modify the dose requirement of the first three shots. BT vaccine also requires a series of shots, which cannot be turned on and off. When is consent to be obtained? And when and how is it necessary to have the field commanders involved?

Second, if there were no penalty for refusal to consent, an incentive would be created on the eve of conflict for individual military personnel to opt out of the obligations they had apparently assumed. If opting out of deployment were allowed, teams that trained together would be impaired, if not destroyed, with attendant loss of military effectiveness. An individual opting out of taking the medication, but being deployed, might place himself or herself at risk and place comrades in jeopardy. Third, strategic considerations might also enter the policy discussion, as discussed in the "not feasible" section above.

Finally, we note that there are certain to be differences between active duty forces and reserve forces for all options but that of seeking consent at time of deployment to a theater of operations in which potential or active conflict exists. We have made no effort to examine those differences here, but they clearly should be examined in the event that consent at recruitment or in basic training are pursued. These differences, in our judgment, argue strongly for consent at time of deployment when the actual nature of risks and benefits are much clearer.

Other Possible Arrangements

Two other options might be considered, neither of which is developed at length here. Their attractiveness would depend on an assessment of the threat of biological warfare and the threat of bioterrorism against U.S. civilian populations. The first possibility would involve the establishment of a "military purposes" category for the review of drugs and vaccines developed for protecting troops who confront the danger of CW/BW agents. The second option would involve a broader "limited purposes" category, which would include "military purposes," but would extend to protecting the civilian population against bioterrorism threats.

A military-purposes approach might be limited to drugs and vaccines developed for responding to military exigencies, such as CW/BW threats, and to endemic infectious diseases in countries to which troops might be deployed. The military may be unique in sending people into danger involuntarily. Public safety personnel, for example, police, fire, or other emergency personnel, always have the option of quitting their jobs. But inherent command authority in the military provides the basis for telling troops to wear their gas masks, to put on their MOPP gear, or to take their pills.

This military-purposes approach would require a rigorous process for evaluating the evidence of safety and efficacy. A critical question is whether the standards of approval for military purposes would be the same as for commercial drug approval purposes. One component of this question is whether human efficacy data are needed for approval. If so, how might they be obtained? If not, what data might be satisfactory as a substitute? Would nonhuman primate challenge data be acceptable? Would surrogate endpoints, such as antibody levels achieved after vaccination, be satisfactory?

A "limited purposes" approach that addressed both military and nonmilitary might also be considered, with nonmilitary referring, for example, to terrorist attacks against U.S. civilian populations. The approach would derive its rationale from an assessment of the threat of bioterrorism and from the reasonable expectation that any organized response involving public health authorities or emergency authorities (e.g., the Federal Emergency Management Agency) would probably confront as much, if not more, confusion as the DoD did in the Gulf War. A limited-purposes approach would allow the addition of categories as the need arose, could impose marketing restrictions, and could require special reporting.

Both the military-purposes and the broader limited-purposes approaches would require extensive public discussion and debate of the issues, including constitutional concerns for "the common defense" and "the general welfare." The discussion would have to lay out relative roles and responsibilities of military and civilian authorities, officials, and agencies, and legislation would undoubtedly be required to establish either and to ensure an adequate legal foundation for administrative behavior.

Chapter Five

BROADER ISSUES

The Request for Comments asked the following questions of a general nature. In our view, these have either been answered or can only be answered in the rule-making process:

- If the interim rule is needed, are there changes that should be made to it based on experiences during and following the Gulf War? If so, what are these changes and why should they be made?

- Can or should the interim rule be narrowed in scope? If so, how?

- Should the rule contain additional procedures to enhance understanding, oversight, and accountability? If so, what are these procedures?

- Are there circumstances under which the use of the interim rule would be justified? If so, what are those circumstances?

In this chapter, we briefly address issues raised by the Interim Rule that are internal to the DoD, some of which affect the external policy issues; we also discuss questions related to DoD-FDA interactions. Finally, we consider "the Question of Authority."

INTERNAL DOD ISSUES

Internal issues associated with the use of investigational drugs for CW/BW defense include training, education, and record keeping, which have been addressed above; integration of external policy into DoD-wide doctrine, policies, and procedures; CW/BW threat analysis; physical availability of drugs and vaccines (inventories of CW/BW countermeasures, drug/vaccine production capabilities, logistics); and the rules for allocation of drugs and vaccines under conditions of scarce supply. These internal issues, which are summarized in Table 3, are of great importance but are beyond the scope of this study. Here we comment briefly only on two issues: integration and threat analysis.

Table 3

Internal DoD Issues of Military Use of Drugs and Vaccines for CW/BW Defense

Primary Issue	Secondary Issues
Integration of medical, operational, and intelligence functions	Incorporating DoD-FDA agreements, including FDA regulations, into DoD doctrine, policies, and procedures for both peacetime and wartime implementation
	Establishing and maintaining DoD effective communication among and between medical, operational, and intelligence entities and authorities
Threat analysis	Routine threat analysis (ongoing, periodic, episodic)
	Crisis threat analysis
	Validation of CW/BW threat and use
	Public understanding of threat
Availability of drugs and vaccines	Budgetary allocations
	Assessment of need (short and long term)
	Development process (long term)
	Licensing policies, procedures, and practices (short, mid, and long term)
	Production (sources, capacity, security)
	Stocks (inventories and shelf life) and storage capabilities
	Logistics
Implementation of actual use	Allocation decisions
	Logistics of administration (capability, supply, allocation criteria, schedule, dosage, discretion of local command authority)
	Information to personnel
	Informed consent
	Record keeping (individuals, units)

The integration of external policies, such as the FDA Interim Rule, into DoD doctrine, policies, and procedures, is a major problem identified in the wake of the Gulf War. This issue has two dimensions: (1) the incorporation of DoD-FDA agreements into DoD doctrine, policy, and procedures during peacetime for implementation in wartime and (2) the establishment of effective communication among and between DoD medical, operational, and intelligence entities and authorities.

The discrepancy between the strictures of the Interim Rule and behaviors of military commanders in the Gulf War highlights the integration problem. The primary communication channel in the formulation of the policy ran from DoD medical, which included the offices of AASD(HA) and the Surgeon General of the Army, to FDA. Communication channels running to the theater of operations led from ASD(HA) to the Joint Staff, and through J-4 to Central Command (Schwarzkopf) and his chief surgeon. No one directly involved in policy formulation was in direct communication with those responsible for implementation. Given that less than one month elapsed between the Interim Rule and the start of hostilities and only one week between the waivers and hostilities and that the U.S. force consisted of nearly 600,000 personnel, it is hardly surprising that communication problems occurred.

The matter of remedies for this internal communication problem is not easy. However, in the discussion below regarding the question of authority, we propose that the Secretary of Defense submit waiver requests, under the Interim Rule or under a modified version of the rule, to the Secretary of Health and Human Services, rather that having ASD(HA) submit them to the FDA Commissioner (see below). The rationale for this proposal is that such a submission route would force internal DoD staffing to address the request that would involve medical, operational, and intelligence activities.

The assessment of worldwide CW/BW threats obviously must be a continuous function. On the other hand, once a thorough assessment of capabilities has been conducted, the primary task is monitoring for changes and anomalies and maintaining intelligence regarding intentions of potential enemies. The appropriate balance between routine and special assessments and short- and long-term assessments is beyond the scope of this report, as is allocation of resources for threat assessment; for a responsive research and development program; and for production, licensing, and logistics capabilities.

One issue that deserves attention in this context is the degree to which threat assessment information is held tightly as secret information or is publicly discussed in open session with Congress and the press. The nuclear threat was widely discussed in the press and before Congress over a period of decades, with confidential information protected in well-established ways. That threat was also the subject of many books and articles in the open literature, with Herman Kahn's *On Thermonuclear War* marking the start of a major public discourse, and the subject of many graduate school courses. One result of this public attention was a public much better informed about nuclear warfare and its prospects and implications than is the case for chemical and biological warfare possibilities. An item on the DoD agenda, then, might be the benefits of a more open discussion for purposes of securing a more informed citizenry and for providing a deeper understanding of the issues underlying such policies as the FDA's Interim Rule.

THE QUESTION OF AUTHORITY

A major issue raised by the controversy over the Interim Rule, but one on which FDA did not ask for comments, is the tension between the inherent authority of the President as Commander in Chief and the authority the FDCA conferred on the FDA. The issue is how to reconcile the legal, ethical, and regulatory requirements of military and civilian authority in actual or potential combat situations in which the threat of chemical and biological warfare agents exists and when the available countermeasures include drugs and vaccines classified as investigational by FDA.

Inherent Command Authority

One of the primary reasons for which the government of the United States was established and the Constitution written was "to provide for the common defense." Article I, Section 8, vests authority in Congress to declare war and raise armies. Article II, Section 2, stipulates that "The President shall be Commander in Chief" of the armed services. Title 10, U.S. Code, pertains to the "Armed Services," and its several parts deal respectively with "organization and general military powers," "personnel"; "training and education"; and "service, supply, and procurement."

In general, command authority as established in the Constitution and by statute is an adequate basis for the conduct of military operations, both in peacetime and in war. This authority extends to requirements of training, uniforms to be worn, relations between officers and enlisted personnel, obligations to protect vital national security information from unauthorized personnel, and many other features of military life. The authority to direct soldiers to take medications or vaccines, to wear a uniform of a certain type, to train to use a particular weapon, although not spelled out in Title 10, U.S. Code, inheres in command authority; detailed applications of that authority exist in a number of Supreme Court cases, as the government's brief in the 1991 Gulf War litigation before the U.S. Court of Appeals makes clear (938 F.2d 1370, No. 91-5019, US App DC 111, July 16, 1991).[1] In active military conflict, command authority

---

[1]The exercise of command authority governs a number of behaviors of military personnel. For example, the *European Stars & Stripes* for May 12, 1997, carried a story by J. P. Barham and Chuck Vinch, "Army sticks it to soldiers: Pierced tongues, noses, soon to be banned," which reported that a planned update of Army Regulation 670-1, pertaining to the wearing of bodily jewelry, would read: "No jewelry, rings, or other devices will be worn or attached to the exposed parts of the body (nose, tongue, lips) except . . . as already permitted by earring guidelines." The implementation of the DoD anthrax vaccination policy also illustrates this point. The July 1, 1998, DoD web site (**http://www.defenselink.mil/other_info/protection.html**) includes the following exchange: Question 39. "Will those refusing to be vaccinated be court-martialed? Discharged?" Answer. "Each case will have to be determined on its own merits but in general persons refusing to comply will face disciplinary action."

conveys great discretion to field commanders, who must make the tactical decisions that implement broad strategic and policy considerations.

One thing made abundantly clear by the Gulf War is that military command authority was not developed with reference to the use of investigational drugs as a defense against CW/BW agents. In actual or potential combat situations that may involve the use of CW/BW agents by an enemy, the military confronts three related needs: to protect individual service members against such agents, to ensure that the behavior of individuals does not jeopardize their immediate fellow soldiers and impair unit integrity, and to maintain an effective war-fighting capability overall. Refusal to consent may cause problems in all three areas. Accomplishing these purposes requires an array of countermeasures against CW/BW threats, including detection equipment, protective clothing and masks, and prophylactic and therapeutic medications. FDA-approved medications pose no problem for military use. Drugs and vaccines classified as investigational also pose no problems if informed consent is obtained from soldiers before they are used and if no penalty attaches to refusal of consent. But when some countermeasures are investigational drugs, and the military concludes that it is not feasible to obtain informed consent for their use, the question arises as to the authority needed for DoD to use such drugs and vaccines.

The Authority of the FDCA

FDCA requirements, as indicated in Chapter One, govern the distribution of licensed drugs in interstate commerce, the conduct of investigations regarding new drugs, and the review and approval of INDs. They are extensive and detailed, as are the informed consent regulations. However, as was true for inherent command authority, the Gulf War made clear that neither FDCA nor its implementing regulations were developed with the use of investigational drugs as a defense against CW/BW agents in mind. Neither had Congress or the courts addressed this issue with explicit statutory directives or judicial interpretations. The Gulf War, then, presented a novel situation for both DoD and FDA, for which the policy question is whether the existing legal, regulatory, and ethical framework is adequate.

Accommodating Military Command Authority and the FDCA

The element of novelty in the current situation is not that public policies developed for one set of purposes conflict with those developed for a different set of purposes. Conflict between independently articulated policies occurs often.

More important, in our judgment, are the mechanisms to accommodate conflicting interests. In the case of DoD and FDA with respect to the development and use of drugs and vaccines, we may identify the following mechanisms that represent accommodation of these different interests.

- First, the MOU, originating in 1964 and last updated in 1987, provides a framework for dealing with DoD's clinical investigation of drugs (52 FR 33472, September 3, 1987). In essence, the MOU is a medical, ethical, and political-military policy declaration that such investigations are to be no different when sponsored or conducted by DoD than when they are sponsored by or performed under the auspices of civilian federal government agencies or private entities subject to federal regulations.

- Second, Sec. 980 requires that informed consent be obtained in all clinical investigations sponsored or conducted by the DoD.

- Third, DoD adherence to FDA regulations for the conduct of clinical investigations involving drugs and vaccines is explicit acknowledgment that the human subjects of those investigations sponsored or conducted by the military are to be treated no differently from the requirements that apply to similar investigations in the civilian sector.

- Fourth, DoD adherence to the Common Rule governing the protection of human subjects [45 CFR 46, Subpart A—Federal Policy for the Protection of Human Subjects (Basic DHHS Policy for Protection of Human Research Subjects)] is explicit acknowledgment that human subjects of investigations sponsored or conducted by the military are to be treated no differently from the requirements that apply to similar investigations in the civilian sector.

- Finally, the Interim Rule represents an FDA response to a DoD request for establishing a mechanism to deal with certain military combat exigencies, in this case the Iraqi threats, unique in recent history, to engage in CW/BW warfare.

The major issue here is the *adequacy* of these mechanisms in the light of the Gulf War experience. Does the MOU between DoD and FDA provide an adequate legal framework for addressing the issues that arose in the Gulf War and that may arise again in similar, though not identical, form in the future? Given that DoD has submitted itself to the informed consent regulations of DHHS (the Common Rule) and FDA (pertaining to drug development), are such regulations adequate for military contingencies that may arise, such as the Gulf War? Since seven full years have elapsed and since FDA, despite some public pressure to act, has yet to complete the rule-making process, this suggests the complexity of the issues surrounding the relation of military command authority and the FDCA.

Two questions from the July 31, 1997, FDA Request for Comments indicate how this conflict of authority arises in the context of that agency's decision to complete rule making:

- Question A.3 asks: "The interim rule is based on the premise that informed consent is not feasible in military combat exigencies because if a soldier were permitted to say 'no,' this could jeopardize the individual soldier's life, endanger other personnel in his or her unit, and jeopardize the accomplishment of the combat mission. DoD has alleged that it is not an option to excuse a nonconsenting solider from a military mission. Given the experience in the Gulf War, does this rationale still hold?"

- Question A.8 (b) asks: "Should the authority to make the "feasibility determination" (i.e., whether obtaining informed consent is "not feasible") under the interim rule be vested in persons or entities other than the Commissioner of FDA?"

The question of whether the FDA Commissioner should make the "not feasible" determination, if answered in the affirmative, opens the door to an involvement of the commissioner in military matters that goes well beyond the authority inherent in FDCA and clearly exceeds the traditional competence of the commissioner. It invites FDA to intrude deeply into military matters in instances similar to the Gulf War. We argue that an FDA that is highly intrusive in military operations is undesirable for the potential constitutional conflict that it may generate. Consequently, our response to the above question is negative: The FDA Commissioner should *not* be the U.S. government official responsible for making the "not feasible" determination.

If answered negatively, however, the question becomes, "If not the FDA Commissioner, then whom?" The answer depends on whether one thinks the issue is a medical or a political-military one. If one accepts the view that the Interim Rule is both a medical and a political-military policy, and that requests for waivers under the rule require both medical and political-military decisions, an argument exists for making decisions at the highest level of political authority— within DHHS, the Secretary, and within DoD, the Secretary of Defense.

This logic opens the door to requests for waiver of informed consent originating with the Secretary of Defense, being transmitted to the Secretary of Health and Human Services, and the determination of "not feasible" being made either by the Secretary of HHS or jointly by the Secretary of HHS and the Secretary of Defense. Such a course would not relieve the FDA of its obligation to review such a request, but it would do so now at the direction of the Secretary of HHS, the highest political authority in the department.

Neither would such a course relieve the ASD(HA), nor the Surgeons General of the military services, of their obligations to assess the threat and to recommend a request for waiver of informed consent. It would require that DoD base a waiver request recommendation on input from medical, operational, and intelligence agencies, including concurrence from the field command. Indeed, it is clear that there was a serious breakdown in the implementation of the Interim Rule in the Gulf War, especially with respect to information provided to the affected military personnel, the training of medical and nonmedical personnel, and record keeping. This breakdown stemmed, in part, we believe, from the fact that a policy seen primarily as medical required for its implementation the active input from both military operations and military intelligence.

Would time permit such a course of action to be followed? In the case of the Gulf War, nearly four months elapsed from the initial discussions of the need for what became the Interim Rule until its issuance. If rule making should result in reissuance in modified form of the Interim Rule, the issue becomes the processing of waiver requests under the rule. It is not clear that staffing for waiver requests with a rule in place would require any more time than it took to issue the Interim Rule in the first place.

The pertinent unresolved concerns about the incomplete accommodation of these two sources of authority in our national life, then, are these. Might a threat similar to what emerged in the Gulf War recur within the foreseeable future and, if it did, would the absence of a clear policy on the use of investigational drugs for CW/BW defense help or hinder the ability of the U.S. government to defend its national interest? If such a threat recurred, would the national interest be best served by having a settled policy or by being forced to make policy in the shadow of war? To answer these questions, it is necessary to address several other issues in greater detail.

A question raised during the fall of 1990 was whether DoD was obligated to submit to FDCA authority for issues related to military combat, such as using investigational drugs for CW/BW defense. Why should DoD not assert the inherent authority of command? This question was informally discussed within DoD, between DoD and FDA, and within DHHS. No definitive answer was forthcoming, because the question was not raised formally, and it remains untested legally and politically.[2]

Some DoD officials thought that it might be sufficient legally to assert inherent command authority without reference to FDCA but that, as a matter of policy, it was better to comply with the FDCA. Others considered the implications of full compliance with FDCA by using investigational drugs with informed consent and complying, or seeking to comply, with all the rest of the IND regulatory requirements. ASD(HA) Mendez took the view that DoD should submit to FDCA authority but should also not represent its action regarding PB and BT as

---

[2]It is possible, however, that the question might be raised again in a slightly different way in the rule-making context at the time of this writing, i.e., under what circumstances might it be appropriate for DoD to act without FDA authorization.

research but as treatment, and therefore, compliance was accompanied by a request to FDA to establish authority to waive informed consent. The Mendez view prevailed and effectively answered the question at a practical level of whether DoD should act independently of FDCA.[3]

If DoD had been unable to obtain the FDA waiver authority of the Interim Rule, and the subsequent waivers for PB and BT, would it have acted on the basis of command authority regarding the use of PB and BT? The scenario response goes something like the following: In all likelihood, the question would have gone from the DoD General Counsel to the Secretary of Defense, who would have consulted the Chairman of the Joint Chiefs of Staff, GEN Colin Powell, and the Commander of Central Command, GEN Norman Schwartzkopf. If in the judgment of the Chairman of the Joint Chiefs and the CENTCOM it had been important to use PB and BT, or to have the authority to do so in the event that these drugs were needed, they would have then responded to the General Counsel with the query, "Can you defend this legally?" The General Counsel would then probably have gone forward with an argument about general command authority in the Constitution and Title 10, U.S. Code, the clarity of Supreme Court case law supporting command authority, and the absence of any "private cause of action" to challenge the FDCA other than by the Commissioner of the FDA. This is the hypothetical case in which DoD would rely exclusively on the authority of the Commander in Chief.

Three factors suggest that the above course of action, though possibly defensible on legal grounds, might have limited utility as a public policy. One consideration was that FDA review of the policy issue and of the specific waivers might benefit the DoD by counterbalancing military medical R&D thinking with an outside, independent view.[4] The second consideration was that a policy that might be legally defensible in time of war might not be politically sustainable in the postwar environment. The controversy surrounding the Gulf War, a short, militarily successful campaign, in the past five years, suggests that this is the case and underlines the importance of closely linking legal authority and political support if policy is to succeed.

The final consideration has to do with the costs, benefits, and risks of taking this kind of an issue to the President for resolution. He is, after all, the ultimate arbiter of disputes between cabinet-level departments and is the Commander in Chief. Such a course of action, however, is not to be considered lightly. The brief for the Secretary of Defense and the Secretary of Health and Human Ser-

---

[3]Interview with John Casciotti.

[4]This construction was provided by one participant who observed that Dr. Enrique Mendez saw FDA involvement as beneficial from the medical viewpoint, while the Office of General Counsel saw it as beneficial from the legal viewpoint.

vices filed in the U.S. Court of Appeals for the District of Columbia Circuit in *Doe v. Sullivan* posed the issue in the following terms:

> Doe's challenge to these actions [i.e., issuance of the Interim Rule and granting of waivers under the rule] is an extraordinary one. It represents an unprecedented attempt by a military serviceman during wartime to judicially countermand decisions by his superiors about the conduct of the war. It asks the courts, in the name of enforcing statutes regarding unapproved drugs, to interfere with the President's constitutional power as Commander-in-Chief to direct the battlefield activities of the armed forces while actually in combat. And it asserts statutory and constitutional claims which, if recognized, may imperil the lives of military personnel and civilians and jeopardize the prosecution of the war. [p. 20]

and later

> if Section 505(I) [of the FDCA] were construed to foreclose DoD from administering investigational drugs for tactical purposes in a combat theater, a grave question would be presented concerning the impact of the statute on the President's constitutional powers as Commander-in-Chief. Whatever the ultimate scope of those powers may be, they clearly encompass the exclusive authority to determine (directly or through the President's subordinates) how a military campaign authorized by Congress is to be carried out in the field. *Cf. Youngstown*, 343 U.S. at 645 (Jackson, J., concurring) (courts "should indulge the widest latitude of interpretation to sustain [the President's] exclusive function to command the instruments of national force"). That authority cannot constitutionally be withdrawn or denied by Congress or the courts. Thus, insofar as Section 505(I) could possibly be construed to limit the President's discretion as Commander-in-Chief concerning the prophylactic use of investigational drugs as a defensive measure on the battlefield, it almost certainly would be a constitutional nullity as applied. Section 505(I) therefore should be construed to avoid the constitutional problems that would be presented by Doe's construction. [pp. 39–40]

Avoiding the potential conflict between inherent command authority and the authority of FDCA should be regarded as an important public policy objective. This leads to the question addressed in the following section: What mechanisms exist by which conflicts between DoD and FDA might be resolved in a Gulf War–like case, short of taking the matter to the President?

INTERACTIONS BETWEEN DOD AND FDA

What is the nature of the continuing DoD-FDA interaction? Is it adequate? Must it be product specific? Or might it be devoted to general issues periodically? How does the MOU provide a framework for interaction? What are the lessons of the Interim Rule?

The laws and regulations of the FDA that pertain to the development of therapeutic products (drugs, biologics, medical devices) have been developed pursuant to the commerce clause of the Constitution for the primary purpose of ensuring that the safety and effectiveness of these products is established before their introduction to the commercial market. Drug regulation originates in the 1906 Pure Food Act, which required that drugs not be misbranded or adulterated; it was extended by the 1938 FDCA, which requires the evaluation of new drugs for safety, and by the 1962 amendments, which require evaluation for effectiveness. Evaluation of biologics originates in the Public Health Service Act (42 USC 262, 263), deriving from the public health nature of vaccine development for the control of infectious diseases. In recent years, evaluation of biologics has also been drawn under the authority of FDCA. Evaluation of medical devices stems from the Medical Device Amendments of 1976 to FDCA (21 USC 351, 352, 360), as later amended.

The FDCA, as it pertains to drug and biologic evaluation, was not written with military drug and vaccine development in mind. This poses no problem as long as military drug development is comparable to civilian drug development for the commercial marketplace. But military drug development differs at times from commercial drug development in several important ways.

First, the purpose of military drug development is essentially similar to civilian drug development for the most part, but it has the additional purpose to develop and use drugs to protect military personnel from threats that are peculiar to military action. The specialized needs of military medicine, e.g., vaccines developed for defense against potential BW agents and for endemic diseases in remote environments, mean that a dual-use (i.e., military and civilian) commercial market does not always exist for a number of the needed products. Consequently, some drugs are likely to remain in the IND status indefinitely, as is also the case for a number of CDC-developed vaccines, because they are unattractive to commercial sponsors who are unwilling to incur the costs of their further development through the licensing stage.

Second, the economics of commercial drug development involve substantial financial and human resource investments in scientific research, clinical trials, and regulatory affairs. The average development time for a new drugs has been 10–12 years at an estimated cost of $350 million or higher per FDA-approved product. Drug development teams are assembled for a new product, teams that provide continuity of attention, depth of knowledge, and a division of labor appropriate to the task of taking a new chemical entity or a new biologic from the IND stage through the NDA licensing stage. Resources to support drug development are derived from debt or equity financing, or from internal allocation of profits from other products, in anticipation of a profit stream that is sustained over the patent life of the drug.

By contrast, military drug development is characterized by less investment in both financial and human resources. Teams are smaller, seldom assigned to a single compound or biologic. Rotation of military personnel characterizes these teams. Fewer resources are devoted to the regulatory affairs side of licensing, as distinct from the aspects of research and clinical trials. Funds are derived from those appropriated to the DoD for research. In a time of declining budgets, which has been true for the past decade for DoD, scarce resources loom large as a constraint on military drug development and are unlikely to allow DoD to pursue licensing aggressively.

Finally, in addition to highly localized threats from endemic infectious diseases, military drug development confronts the threat of chemical and biological warfare more directly in the wake of the Gulf War than at any other time since World War I. The scientific and clinical problem, then, is not restricted to developing a drug or vaccine for use against a given disease conditions, but embraces the development of drugs for prophylactic purposes against lethal agents deployed by an enemy.

It is this emergence of the CW/BW threat that argues against a simplistic assumption that military drug development can be compared to civilian, commercial drug development. The decades-long process by which FDCA regulations were articulated through the Notice and Comment procedures required by the Administrative Procedures Act, with responses to proposed rules provided by a very large, very profitable, very powerful commercial pharmaceutical industry, does not provide a model for the development of policies related to military drug development in the face of CW/BW threats.

In the spring of 1991, after hostilities in the Gulf War had ended, ASD(HA), Dr. Enrique Mendez, wrote the Director of the Joint Staff of DoD regarding the use of the informed consent waiver for "specific Investigational New Drugs" in the Gulf War about the merit of "a formalization of the FDA approval process." His senior staff, he reported, had taken steps "to define the requirements for informed consent, and the utilization of investigational drugs, devices, and vaccines." Prior FDA approval, he noted, would provide "a responsive mechanism" for the use of investigational products in a military contingency. "Therefore," he wrote,

> we plan to conduct an *annual meeting* [emphasis added] of appropriate representatives from DoD and FDA to review, identify and obtain contingency FDA approval of investigational products of specific military interest.

Mendez may have overreached in his aspirations. FDA prefers, by reason of long-established custom, to deal with general issues in the context of rule making and to address specific issues in the context of reviewing specific IND and NDA applications. They argue, appropriately regarding the latter, that questions of safety and effectiveness, language about labeling, etc., can best be addressed with reference to specific proposals. Nothing has come of the annual meeting proposal.

However, some current interaction along the Mendez lines suggested has occurred. Specifically, a meeting of the CBER anti-virals advisory committee was held in 1996 to review with DoD representatives the studies that would be necessary for DoD to obtain licensing approval for BT vaccine. DoD is currently at work seeking to respond to the advice it received.

Importantly, FDA Deputy Commissioner Mary Pendergast, in testimony to PAC on July 29, 1997, indicated how the agency intended to proceed in rule making. Based on the information received in response to the Request for Comments, she stated, FDA may decide "to hold an open public meeting on a more limited subset of issues." Such a meeting would later be followed by publication of an NPRM. She then added: "Because of the complexity and controversial nature of the issues involved, it will be incumbent on the agency to forge consensus with [sic] the executive branch prior to taking final action."

It would be prudent for DoD to add its collective support for such a public meeting, even to endorse a joint meeting, to seek to assist in defining the issues to be considered, either by negotiation with FDA or by formal submissions to it, and to participate fully in the meeting. Although such a meeting, if held, will focus on issues associated with the Interim Rule, it might facilitate movement toward a regular annual meeting between DoD and FDA on general issues not addressed in rule making and broader than the specific issues of a particular IND or NDA application.

The main point of this section, in summary, is to suggest strongly that a more public and systematic mechanism of interaction is needed between DoD and FDA with respect to the special problems of military drug development than currently exists. The above analysis points to this conclusion.

Chapter Six

CONCLUSIONS AND RECOMMENDATIONS

On the basis of the foregoing analysis, we reached the following conclusions about the policy governing the use of investigational drugs by DoD for certain military combat exigencies. First, although policymaking in the shadow of war may involve careful deliberation, as occurred in the months preceding the Gulf War, it is better to have an adequate policy in place beforehand, broad enough to respond to a number of contingencies and yet narrow enough to avoid abuse or confusion.

Second, as preliminary orienting assumptions to the regulatory regime, it is important to recognize that the threat of CW/BW agents being used against U.S. military forces has permanently altered the context in which the use of investigational drugs is being considered. In addition, notwithstanding many similarities, there are important differences between military drug development and commercial drug development for a civilian market.

Third, a rule authorizing the Commissioner of FDA to waive informed consent for the use of investigational drugs in certain military situations is needed. The Interim Rule provided an adequate policy in the Gulf War, notwithstanding major problems in its implementation. A modification of this rule is likely to result from the completion of rule making. However, complete revocation of the existing rule could be potentially very dangerous in operational terms if it limited DoD's ability to respond to CW/BW threats.

Fourth, *investigational* is a term without precise meaning. It does not demarcate the boundary between research and treatment with a bright orange line. Rather, it constitutes a gray zone in which most of the activity is research, much of the activity involves both research and treatment, and some activity is solely treatment.

Fifth, the most sensible modifications of the current Interim Rule would involve briefly indicating the general requirements for the provision of information to military personnel, training of medics and others responsible for administration of vaccines, training of commanders responsible for ordering self-administration of drugs, and record keeping. The detailed requirements that might apply in any given situation should be developed at the time of a specific waiver request application.

Sixth, the ethical issue regarding informed consent involves a conflict between a view whose priority is the protection of human subjects against the risks of research and one whose priority is the protection of individual military personnel from the risks of lethal chemical and/or biological agents at the price of overriding autonomy.

Seventh, issues internal to DoD that require attention are the integration of the medical, operational, and intelligence aspects associated with the use of investigational drugs when confronting CW/BW threats. To facilitate this integration, and on the assumption that a rule similar to the Interim Rule is adopted, the recommendation is made that the request for waivers under such a rule be submitted by the Secretary of Defense to the Secretary of Health and Human Services, rather than by the ASD(HA) to the FDA Commissioner. This will force internal DoD attention to the use of investigational drugs by all parties concerned, not just by the medical arm of the department.

Eighth, a Constitutional conflict between inherent command authority and the authority of the FDCA exists as a possibility in the absence of a settled policy on the use of investigational issues. Such a conflict is to be avoided if at all possible, and this objective should inform policy development. Several recommendations have been made in the report to anticipate and eliminate this potential conflict.

Finally, a process of continual interaction between DoD and FDA is needed. Military drug development shares many features with civilian drug development for commercial purposes, but it also has distinct characteristics. Recognition of these distinct characteristics leads to the recommendation that a venue be found, perhaps an annual DoD-FDA conference on "issues in military drug development," that deals with general issues not amenable to rule making and broader than those considered in a specific IND or NDA application.

Chapter Seven

POSTSCRIPT

In July 1997, as indicated above, FDA issued "Accessibility to New Drugs for Use in Military and Civilian Exigencies When Traditional Human Efficacy Studies Are Not Feasible; Determination Under the Interim Rule That Informed Consent is Not Feasible for Military Exigencies; Request for Comments," (62 FR 40996, July 31, 1997). This request asked for public comment on issuing the Interim Rule unchanged as a final rule, modifying the rule, or revoking it.

It was anticipated at the time of the Request for Comments that this action would subsequently result in an FDA proposed decision, which in turn would be published as an NPRM. Formal publication of an NPRM had not occurred by the summer of 1998, although it was known that FDA had submitted to OMB for clearance a proposal (i.e., a draft NPRM) to revoke the Interim Rule. This proposal was not a public document. It was also known, although not formally public, that DoD had objected to revocation.

During the summer of 1998, the "Bryd amendment" (S. 2057, July 20, 1998) was included in the Senate national defense authorization bill for fiscal year 1999. This amendment would have removed the authority to submit *waiver requests* under the Interim Rule from ASD(HA) and vested that authority in the Secretary of Defense. The proposed amendment further required that the President concur in this request, by a written statement, and that the chairman and ranking minority member of each "congressional defense committee" be notified of this action. If enacted, however, the amendment required that the Interim Rule, or its equivalent, authorizing such waivers continue in effect. Given the FDA proposal to revoke the Interim Rule, the possibility existed briefly, and perhaps only hypothetically, that a statute would be enacted authorizing the Secretary of Defense to request implementation of a nonexistent FDA regulation.

The Gordian knot was cut in a modified version of the Byrd amendment, included as Sec. 731 of the Strom Thurmond National Defense Authorization Act for Fiscal Year 1999 (Public Law 105-261, October 17, 1998). This amendment, entitled "Process for Waiving Informed Consent Requirement for Administration of Certain Drugs to Members of Armed Forces for Purposes of a Particular Military Operation," pertained to "the administration of an investigational new drug or a drug unapproved for its applied use to a member of the armed forces in connection with the member's participation in a particular military operation." It provided that the requirement of prior consent for receipt of such a drug under the FDCA "may be waived only by the President."

The President, in granting waivers under this provision, must determine in writing "that obtaining consent—(A) is not feasible; (B) is contrary to the best interests of the member; or (C) is not in the interests of national security." In reaching such a determination, the President "shall apply the standards and criteria that are set forth in the relevant FDA regulations for a waiver of the prior consent requirement on that ground." The relevant FDA regulations are specified as those "promulgated under section 505(i) of the FDCA; the prior consent requirements are those specified under section 505(i)(4)." The notification of the Committee on Armed Services and the Committee on Appropriations of the Senate, and the Committee on National Security and the Committee on Appropriations of the House of Representatives are required of any waivers granted under this provision.

Thus, the issue of authority has been decisively resolved. The granting of waivers of informed consent is now, by statute, recognized as not only a scientific and clinical issue, but one that requires the engagement of the highest political authority under the Constitution, the President of the United States, with full knowledge of the relevant congressional committees. The defense against CW/BW weapons of mass destruction has thus been elevated to the level of the Commander in Chief. Questions of implementation now must be clarified. Presumably, issues of dealing with chemical and biological terrorism will now also engage Presidential authority.

21 *Code of Federal Regulations* §312.110, Miscellaneous, 1991.

21 *Code of Federal Regulations* §312.34, "Treatment Use of an Investigational New Drug," 1991.

21 *Code of Federal Regulations* §50, "Protection of Human Subjects," 1991.

52 *Federal Register* 33472, "Memorandum of Understanding Between the Department of Defense and the Food and Drug Administration," September 3, 1987.

55 *Federal Register* 52814, "Informed Consent for Human Drugs and Biologics; Determination That Informed Consent is Not Feasible," December 21, 1990.

62 *Federal Register* 40996, "Accessibility to New Drugs for Use in Military and Civilian Exigencies When Traditional Human Efficacy Studies Are Not Feasible; Determination Under the Interim Rule That Informed Consent is Not Feasible for Military Exigencies; Request for Comments," July 31, 1997.

Advisory Committee on Human Radiation Experiments, *The Human Radiation Experiments: Final Report of the Presidential Advisory Committee,* New York, Oxford University Press, 1996.

Annas, G. J., "Changing the Consent Rules for Desert Storm," *New England Journal of Medicine,* No. 326, 1992, pp. 770–773.

Annas, G., and M. A. Grodin, Commentary on "Treating the Troops" by EG Howe and ED Martin, *Hastings Center Report,* Vol. 21, No. 2, 1991, pp. 24–27.

Annas, G., and M. A. Grodin, *The Nazi Doctors and the Nuremberg Code,* New York: Oxford University Press, 1992.

Caplan, A., Testimony, U.S. Senate, Committee on Veterans' Affairs, "Is Military Research Hazardous to Veterans' Health? Lessons from World War II, the Persian Gulf, and Today," Hearing, May 6, 1994.

Department of Defense, Memorandum to FDA General Counsel, "Medical Products Under IND Regulations Which Are Required or Are Under Consideration for Deployment in Support of Operation Desert Shield," August 31, 1990.

Dunn, M. A., and F. R. Sidell, "Progress in Medical Defense Against Nerve Agents," *Journal of the American Medical Association*, No. 262, 1989, pp. 649–652.

Edgar, H., and D. J. Rothman, "The Institutional Review Board and Beyond: Future Challenges to the Ethics of Human Experimentation," *The Milbank Quarterly*, Vol. 73, No. 4, 1995, pp. 489–506.

Fox, R. C., and J. P. Swazey, *The Courage to Fail: A Social View of Organ Transplants and Dialysis*, 2nd ed., rev., Chicago: University of Chicago Press, 1978.

Gilliat, Robert L., Memorandum for the Assistant Secretary of Defense (Health Affairs), "Applicability of Human Subject Research Restrictions to Potential Medical Treatments in Connection with Operation Desert Shield," September 14, 1990.

Howe, E. G. and E. D. Martin, "Treating the Troops," *Hastings Center Report*, Vol. 21, No. 2, 1991, pp. 21–24.

Informed Consent Waiver Review Group (ICWRG), Memorandum to Commissioner of Food and Drugs, re IND 23,509—Pyridostigmine Bromide 30 mg Tablets—ACTION.

Journal of the American Medical Association, Vol. 276, November 27, 1996. This issue contained seven contributions related to the Nuremberg Code.

Keeler, J. R., C. G. Hurst, M. A. Dunn, "Pyridostigmine Used as a Nerve Agent Pretreatment Under Wartime Conditions," *Journal of the American Medical Association*, No. 266, 1991, pp. 693–695.

Kennedy, Sen. Edward M., Remarks, *Congressional Record*, October 2, 1972, p. S-33154-5.

Lehman, Craig R. (Lt Col, USAF), Memorandum for Record, Proceedings of Meeting Between FDA and DOD Regarding Operation Desert Shield, *Federal Register*, August 30, 1990.

Levine, R. J., Commentary on "Treating the Troops" by EG Howe and ED Martin, *Hastings Center Report*, Vol. 21, No. 2, 1991, pp. 27–29.

Martin, E., Testimony, U.S. Senate, Committee on Veterans Affairs, Is Military Research Hazardous to Veterans' Health? Lessons from World War II, the Persian Gulf, and Today, 103rd Congress, 2nd Session, May 6, 1994, p. 124.

Mendez, Enrique, Jr., M.D., letter to David A. Kessler, M.D., regarding pentavalent botulinum toxoid, December 28, 1990a.

Mendez, Enrique, Jr., M.D., letter to David A. Kessler, M.D., regarding pyridostigmine bromide, December 28, 1990b.

Memorandum from Richard A. Merrill, February 24, 1998

National Commission for the Protection of Human Subjects of Biomedical and Behavioral Research, *The Belmont Report: Ethical Principles and Guidelines for the Protection of Human Subjects of Research*, Office of the Secretary, Department of Health, Education, and Welfare, April 18, 1979. Also 44 *Federal Register* 23193, April 18, 1979.

Nuremberg Code, *Journal of the American Medical Association*, No. 276, 1996, p. 1691.

PAC–*see* Presidential Advisory Committee on Gulf War Veterans' Illnesses.

Pechura, C. M., and D. P. Rall, eds., Institute of Medicine, *Veterans at Risk: The Health Effects of Mustard Gas and Lewisite*, Washington, D.C.: National Academy Press, 1993.

Pendergast, M. K., Statement by Mary K. Pendergast, Deputy Commissioner and Senior Advisor to the Commissioner, Food and Drug Administration, Department of Health and Human Services, before the Presidential Advisory Committee on Gulf War Veterans Illnesses, July 29, 1997.

Persian Gulf Veterans Coordinating Board, Response to the Presidential Advisory Committee on Gulf War Veterans' Illnesses, March 7, 1997.

Presidential Advisory Committee on Gulf War Veterans' Illnesses, Transcript of January 12, 1996a.

Presidential Advisory Committee on Gulf War Veterans' Illnesses, *Interim Report*, February 1996b.

Presidential Advisory Committee on Gulf War Veterans' Illnesses, *Final Report*, December 1996c.

Rettig, R. A., L. E. Earley, and R. A. Merrill, eds., Institute of Medicine, *Food and Drug Administration Advisory Committees*, Washington, D.C.: National Academy Press, 1992.

Robertson, J., "Legal Implications of the Boundaries Between Biomedical Research Involving Human Subjects and the Accepted or Routine Practice of Medicine," in National Commission for the Protection of Human Subjects of Biomedical and Behavioral Research, *The Belmont Report: Ethical Principles and Guidelines for the Protection of Human Subjects of Research*, Appendix

16, Vol. II, Washington, D.C.: Office of the Secretary, Department of Health, Education, and Welfare, April 18, 1979.

Sabiston, D., "The Boundaries Between Biomedical Research Involving Human Subjects and the Accepted or Routine Practice of Medicine, with Particular Emphasis on Innovation in the Practice of Surgery," in National Commission for the Protection of Human Subjects of Biomedical and Behavioral Research, *The Belmont Report: Ethical Principles and Guidelines for the Protection of Human Subjects of Research*, Appendix 17, Vol. II, Washington, D.C.: Office of the Secretary, Department of Health, Education, and Welfare, April 18, 1979.

Scales, R.H., Jr., *Certain Victory: United States Army in the Gulf War*, Washington, D.C.: Office of the Chief of Staff, United States Army, 1993.

Schuchardt, E. J., "Distinguishing Between Research and Medical Practice During Operation Desert Storm, *Food and Drug Law Journal*, No. 49, 1994, pp. 271–289.

Sidell, Takafuji, and Franz, 1997.)

Sisson, George H., Memorandum for Record, "Meeting with FDA, Friday, 14 September 1990," 17 September 1990.

U.S. Court of Appeals for the District of Columbia Circuit. John Doe and Mary Doe, Appellees. July 16, 1991. 938 F.2d 1370; 1991 U.S. App. LEXIS 14984; 291 U.S. App. D.C. 111.

U.S. Department of Defense, Defense Science Board, *Report of the Defense Science Board on Persian Gulf War Health Effects*, June 1994.

U.S. Department of Defense, Protection of Human Subjects in DoD-Supported Research, DoD Directive 3216.2, January 7, 1983.

U.S. District Court for the District of Columbia. John Doe and Mary Doe, Plaintiffs, v. Louis W. Sullivan and Richard Cheney, Defendants. January 31, 1991. 756 F. Supp. 12; 1991 U.S. Dist. LEXIS 1702.

U.S. House of Representatives, Committee on Government Reform and Oversight, Subcommittee on Human Resources, Oversight of HHS: Bioethics and the Adequacy of Informed Consent, Hearing, May 8, 1997.

World Medical Association, Declaration of Helsinki, "Recommendations Guiding Physicians in Biomedical Research Involving Human Subjects," *Journal of the American Medical Association* , No. 277, 1997, pp. 925–926.